Dedication

This book is dedicated to my parents, wife and family. It is also dedicated to all of the researchers and doctors who had the guts and integrity to put our health and well being ahead of profits. Special thanks to the crew at Blodget Publishing; Britney, Donald, Tanya, Tresea and Wanda!

Support

Please take a stand and give this book a positive review if you believe in the message and find the book helpful.

Title and Copyright Page

Hello Health, Goodbye Diets:

How to Reject the American Diet and Eat Whole Foods

About the author

Clifford Blodget has a BS degree in computer science and worked as a research engineer and Technology Officer. Cliff brings a systematic and fact based approach to diets and nutrition, using the latest research and large scale studies to cut through the misinformation and confusion that surround this field. For three generations Cliff's family has been focused on health and nutrition. His parents are academics and have been researching nutrition for over 50 years, many of the ideas and strategies in this book for implementing a whole food diet came from them.

Table of Contents

1 - Getting Started...4

2 - Why The American Diet is Killing Us.............................12

3 - Making The Change...22

4 - Nutritional Foundation for Optimum Health.................31

5 - A Look at Whole Foods..44

6 - Shopping & Grocery Lists...57

7 - Cooking & Preparation..66

8 - Breakfast...82

9 - Lunch & Dinner..89

10 - Exercise & Fitness..109

11 - Nutrition Software...122

12 - Links to Resources & The Fight To Change An Industry.......................126

13 - Jumpstart Meal Plans...135

IMPORTANT NOTICE:

This book is not meant to substitute for medical advice from your doctor. If you have a medical condition or are taking drugs or medication, you should consult your doctor before making changes to your diet or exercise routine. The information in this book is believed to be correct at the time it was written, advances in nutritional science, diets and exercise are being made on a continuous basis, you should always seek new information as it becomes available.

1 - Getting Started

This book is for everyone from competition athletes to office workers, from kids to seniors. If you are tired of weight gain and health problems this is your permanent ticket out. Vital and life changing information is presented about diet and nutrition based on the latest large scale scientific studies. This information contradicts many commonly accepted beliefs, therefore it is important to keep an open mind. I had many of my own misconceptions shattered during the five years of research for this book.

A permanent and flexible way of eating is described that will provide the best long term health possible. It is the way of eating that is at our core nutritionally, anatomically and historically. Eating this way will eliminate weight problems and reduce or eliminate many types of diseases including heart disease, diabetes, erectile dysfunction and most forms of cancer. You will lose weight rapidly if you are overweight and achieve your natural lean weight. Say hello to health and goodbye to dieting!

Jumpstart meal plans

Making a permanent change to your diet can take some time. If you want to get started immediately, you can use the jumpstart meal plans in chapter 13. These nutritionally balanced meal plans can be used as a starting point for your transition to a whole food diet, or they can be used for rapid weight loss. This will allow you to start benefiting while you are reading the book. Unlike fad diets, the jumpstart meal plans are nutritionally complete.

Whole food vs Processed food

Whole food is natural food as it was grown and harvested from plants and trees. Examples of whole foods are cabbage, apples, oranges, beans, nuts, seeds, berries and potatoes. Whole foods are grown, not made in a factory. They do not contain synthetic ingredients such as preservatives, hormones, chemicals, antibiotics, flavor enhancers and artificial food colorings.

Throughout history humans have eaten a whole food diet with modest amounts of lean meat. Our digestive and metabolic systems are specifically optimized for whole foods. During the last 70 years, processed foods and factory farmed animal products have replaced whole foods as the primary foods of the American diet. Meat and dairy consumption has more than doubled and in some cases is many times higher.

Why does this matter? It matters because your body is not made to use processed food and factory farmed animal products. The human digestive system was formed many thousands of years before the existence of processed food. Processed food is unnatural and causes your body to malfunction. For example your metabolic system can't properly regulate your weight resulting in chronic weight gain.

Processed food is broken food, literally. During processing the structure of the food is broken down into parts by machines. Some of the most nutritional parts are discarded. Typically, high temperatures are used and chemicals are added. If this sounds unnatural, you're right. Most of the nutritional value of the food is destroyed during processing and the energy density of the food is increased. Even a small increase in energy density is enough to cause a major increase in your body weight. In chapter two we will cover what processing does to food and why it causes weight gain in more detail.

Processed food and factory farmed animal products are nutritionally deficient and contain toxins that damage the immune system and promote diseases such as heart disease, diabetes, erectile dysfunction and cancer. The damage happens slowly over a long period of time, so most people are not aware that it is happening. Day by day like clockwork, as you eat processed foods and factory farmed animal products your immunity weakens and your body becomes more susceptible to disease.

Wild animals eat whole foods. Have you ever seen an obese wild animal? Seriously, out of all the birds, squirrels, deer or raccoons you have seen, have you ever seen an obese one? Actually, a telling thought is that raccoons and squirrels that live around people and eat food from garbage cans, do get obese and have the same diet related diseases that most Americans have!

Before industrialization it was rare to see obesity in humans. Only wealthy people were obese because wealthy people could afford pastries and cakes with refined sugar and fat. Historically obesity was known as the disease of kings and queens, a disease of affluence. In modern times processed food has expanded from pastries and cakes and now includes most food in the grocery store. Many types of processed foods are deceptively marketed as "healthy" or "natural". The consumption of processed food is so widespread that some people have little or no whole foods in their diet at all. Most people think that the American diet is normal, but from a historical and biological standpoint the American diet is highly abnormal and unhealthy.

A whole food diet excludes processed food and consists only of whole and unbroken food. High quality lean meat is acceptable in limited amounts, but factory farmed meat is avoided because factory farmed meat is considered a processed food (because of what the animals are fed).

Whole foods are high in nutrients and provide the full range of nutrients that your body needs. This range of nutrients can't be provided by vitamins or supplements. Large scale scientific studies and health data show that a whole food diet results in superior health with a huge reduction of diseases such as heart disease, cancer, diabetes, Alzheimer's, and autoimmune disease. These studies and the benefits of a whole food diet are covered in chapter four.

History is repeating itself

The food industry is following the same path that the tobacco industry once traveled. We can learn from history. Sixty years ago almost half of all Americans smoked cigarettes. The effects were devastating, millions of people died from cancer and other diseases caused by smoking. Now smoking is down to 18% of the population and dropping. This decline is the result of hard data showing that smoking promotes cancer and disease.

Today over 75% of all Americans eat a diet comprised mostly of processed food and factory farmed animal products. The effects of the American diet are devastating, millions of people are suffering and dying from heart disease, cancer, diabetes and other diseases. More than 33% of Americans are obese and 70% are overweight.

At first people rejected the data showing the dangers of smoking because smoking is addictive and was perceived as being cool. As the death toll continued to rise, people began taking the situation seriously. Governments finally acted to reduce smoking and make tobacco companies take responsibility for their products. It is now common knowledge that smoking is bad. People that smoke are now perceived as being suicidal or ignorant.

Similarly, although the data clearly shows the dangers of the American diet, most people are continuing to eat processed foods and factory farmed animal products because they are addictive and are advertised as being healthy and desirable. Like the tobacco industry once did, the food industry is doing everything in it's power to deny the health impacts and keep people buying their products. As people continue to gain weight and the death toll rises, more people will take the situation seriously. As we did with smoking, fifty years from now we will look back in disbelief and wonder how anyone could have eaten the American diet.

To protect their interests, the tobacco companies engaged in deceit, including lying to congress and setting up special interest groups to promote misinformation about the dangers of smoking. They went as far as employing scientists to generate fraudulent studies showing that smoking was healthy and casting doubt over legitimate research. These techniques worked to confuse the public and delay government action for many years, but eventually the truth prevailed.

The food industry has learned from the tobacco industry, its techniques are similar but have become more sophisticated. This explains the large amount of misinformation flooding the market about food. They know that people are only capable of processing a limited amount of information and that if they put out massive amounts of conflicting information people will be confused and vulnerable. It takes years of research to sort through this information and get a clear picture, few people actually have the time and resources to do this. Without solid and reliable information most of us will make emotionally based purchasing decisions driven by advertising. This is exactly what the food industry wants us to do.

Popular diets

What about the diets that are popular nowadays? Instead of focusing on the foods that your body needs, some popular diets demonize specific types of foods that are claimed to be bad, like wheat, fat, gluten, dairy, carbohydrates or red meat. This caters to people's desire to scapegoat a bad food but otherwise continue without making a major change to their diet. Unfortunately this approach does not work, because there is no single culprit. The problem with the American diet is caused by many types of foods and by the factory processing of food. Only by rejecting the entire American diet can you control your weight and maintain your health.

Conversely, other popular diets attribute inflated nutritional qualities to certain foods and advocate consuming large quantities of these foods. Juice diets and high protein diets are examples of this. These diets cater to people's desire to embrace something perceived as being good, something that they hope will protect them or make them strong. Focusing on single types of foods is not the answer. These diets are unbalanced and unhealthy, they are not what your body was designed for.

Most popular diets incorporate a social or personal identity aspect. This can be a positive thing for motivation, but can foster an us-against-them mentality. This type of mentality destroys the chance of productive dialog and sharing of information between people, it gets in the way of making rational and fact based decisions about diet and food selection.

What makes this book different

What makes this book different from other books is the focus on how to actually implement a whole food diet. While it is important to understand the science of a whole food diet and the problems of the modern American diet, how to prepare and cook whole foods in a flexible manner needs to be adequately addressed. This seems simple, but it is the primary reason why most people who try to adopt a whole food diet fall short. This book explains how to prepare and cook with whole foods in such a way that anyone, even with little or no cooking experience can make the transition. Exotic foods and ingredients are not used, you will be surprised at how inexpensive a whole food diet can be!

A special feature of this book is the cooking style that is used. Most of the meals are made from side dishes instead of an entree or main course. This gets you going without complicated recipes and is similar to the way that people cook and prepare meals in everyday life. You will be able to whip up many types of meals quickly and easily. Complicated recipes are tedious and most cookbooks sit on the shelf for a good reason. Who has the time to buy long lists of strange ingredients? Who has the time to cook complicated recipes? I sure don't.

The goal of this book is to be as short and readable as possible for a broad cross section of readers. For this reason, extensive references are not listed. References would have added about 75 pages to the length of the book and substantially increased the cost. If you are interested in references, chapter twelve has a list of books with references and links to the peer reviewed research that was used as the basis for this book.

Genetics

Contrary to popular belief genetics are not a significant risk factor for most people. The primary risk factor is our diet. The second is exercise and lifestyle. The third is environmental and occupational exposure. A good way to think about this is that genetics may load the gun, but it takes a bad diet, lifestyle or chemical exposure to pull the trigger. This means that with a healthy diet and exercise most people have a very small chance of getting diseases such as heart disease, cancer, diabetes, Alzheimer's, autoimmune diseases, erectile dysfunction or obesity. You have control. If you adopt a whole food diet and a good exercise program you can avoid being a victim in most cases and have a happier and more productive life.

Why should I change?

Often I hear people say "Yes, but my grandfather lived to be ninety and he was healthy. He ate whatever he wanted to, why should I change my diet?". This is a common argument, but it's wrong because it's based on an exception. Are you willing to gamble your life on being an exception? Eating a modern American diet is like playing Russian roulette with your health which is crazy in my book (no pun intended!). The fact that everybody is doing it does not make it any less crazy.

The reciprocal of the argument above is "I know someone with a perfect diet and they got cancer anyway. Why should I change my diet?" There are other causes of cancer such as air pollution, smoking and occupational exposure. Just because you can get cancer from one of these other factors does not mean you should give up on your diet. A better idea is to minimize your risk from all known factors and stay healthy!

Addiction

Addiction is a bad word and no one likes to think that they have an addiction, but we are all programmed from birth with some level of food addiction. This serves a natural and healthy purpose when we have the whole food diet we were designed to eat, but when we eat processed foods with high levels of sugar, fat and salt these addictions escalate and become very serious. Food addictions are difficult to break, perhaps harder than a drug addiction. This is a contributing factor in the modern obesity epidemic. In chapter three we will cover making the change and breaking food addictions.

The results

Once we are eating whole foods and getting proper exercise most people see significant results:

- Your body will automatically adjust to your optimal weight with no need to diet. Genetic or medical conditions that cause obesity are extremely rare, it's usually the diet.

- Greatly increased levels of long term energy.

- No roller-coaster effect, such as sudden bursts of energy or sudden bouts of sleepiness after eating. You will not "hit the wall" during exercise or have hunger attacks during the day.

- Decreased blood pressure and reduced cholesterol levels.

- Most digestive issues will be a thing of the past, including irritable bowel issues and constipation.

- Most health problems will disappear or become less serious. Even serious diseases like heart disease, cancer, erectile dysfunction and diabetes can be stopped or reversed in most people.

- Most skin problems will be reduced or disappear including acne.

- Fewer headaches, because blood sugar levels are more stable.

- Stress and mood swings will decrease, psychological health will improve.

- Most sleep problems and insomnia will disappear.

- Dental health will improve.

- Quite surprisingly most people will find that their monthly food costs go down when they eat whole foods. Yes, it actually costs less to eat healthy!

Frequently Asked Questions

Question: Where is the bibliography or references?
Answer: Chapter 12 has a comprehensive list of information sources.
Question: Health food is so expensive, I can't afford to change my diet. Any ideas?
Answer: The "Health food" that is sold in the health food section of most grocery stores is not the same as whole food. Health food is generally a reformulated version of regular processed food. For example health food puffed wheat cereal is still a processed food but is formulated with less sugar so it is slightly healthier than regular puffed wheat cereal. For not adding sugar they charge a higher price! Many whole foods on the other hand, can be purchased in the bulk food section of the store to reduce costs. Buy whole food, not "health food". There are other ways to reduce food costs that will be covered in chapter six. Most people are able to reduce their food expense with a whole food diet.

Question: Is this a Vegetarian or Vegan diet?

Answer: No or yes! This diet is a flexible whole food diet. Meat, fish and eggs can be included in reduced quantities or not included at all, the choice is yours. Most of the benefit of a whole food diet is possible with limited meat consumption. This is discussed in chapter five.

Question: Is this a paleo diet?

Answer: No, this differs from paleo in several important ways. Paleo is a high animal protein diet (high consumption of meat and eggs) based on assumptions about what our ancestors ate during the paleolithic period. Modern scientific analysis of bone and teeth samples from paleolithic people show that most of these assumptions are incorrect. For example the assumption that grains and legumes were not eaten during the paleolithic period, and that large quantities of meat were consumed by the majority of paleolithic people have been proven incorrect. This is discussed further in chapter four. Paleo has fragmented and some versions are now more moderate. A good aspect that paleo has in common with a whole food diet is the rejection of processed foods, dairy and the American diet.

Question: I have a pretty good diet, but I can't lose weight. What could be the problem?

Answer: Many people become frustrated and think that they are genetically disposed to being overweight, but usually this is not the case. Eliminate all processed food and factory farmed animal products and your weight will drop. Everyone knows to avoid sugar, but most people are not aware that oil is a processed food with more than double the energy level of pure sugar! Oil is in many foods such as margarine and salad dressings. Vegetable based oils may not directly cause heart disease, but they have no significant nutritional value and are not a necessary part of your diet. Oil has empty calories and causes weight gain. Most bread and baked goods also have a high energy level and should be avoided. If you are going to lose weight and then maintain your natural lean weight, all processed foods must be eliminated.

Question: Why is such a drastic change of diet needed?

Answer: The American diet is not our natural diet. Since the beginning of our species humans have eaten a whole food diet. Completely rejecting the modern American diet is the only way to reclaim our health and wellbeing. No amount of supplements or medications can make the American diet healthy. Partially rejecting the American diet will give you a partial improvement, such as a partial reduction of disease and a partial reduction in obesity. If you want a drastic improvement in health and a permanent reduction in weight, a drastic change of diet is needed.

Question: Should I go through cleansing or detox before starting this diet?

Answer: No. Once you are eating correctly your body will automatically detox itself and will continue to detox itself as long as you are eating healthy. Cleansing and detox products are marketed to make money and are unneeded with a whole food diet.

Question: What you're saying goes against most of what I hear on television and in advertising, how can it be true?

Answer: The food industry and supplement industry are not your friends, they sell products using misinformation and deception. Make no mistake, these industries are in business to maximize profit and sell products, they are not in business to care about your health. You must take control of your health and stop listening to advertising, fads and commonly accepted myths about food and health.

Question: If I make a major change in my diet it will alienate my friends and family.

Answer: Yes, sometimes it will. Be prepared to be different, and try not to be defensive about it. You may receive pressure to conform from the people around you. Most of us are surrounded by people with a standard American diet. They may try to hold you back. Have perseverance, you can overcome this. Try to be positive and set a good example. Never preach. Eventually (and sometimes years later) they may change their diets as well.

Question: Why are people so bitter and polarized when it comes to diets? Why are they so stuck in their ways?

Answer: Because it is tough to be on the wrong side of history. It is tough to learn that everything they thought they knew is wrong. People don't like to admit they are wrong. People in the food industry don't want to think that the hard work that they put in to build products is really hurting people. Many people become bitter and go into denial.

Question: What is it like to exclusively eat whole foods?

Answer: Its great! First of all you can eat as much as you want without weight gain (as long as you are eating balanced meals and not straight peanut butter!). You will never go hungry. In fact because whole foods take longer to digest they provide time released energy for many hours. Even if you miss a meal you won't get very hungry. Your long term energy level will be high and you won't "hit the wall" or have a dip in energy after 30 minutes when exercising. Most people stop getting the flu. It is common for people with whole food diets to need no medication. It is a marvel to watch the body take care of itself and do what it was designed to do. After adjusting to whole foods, you will find that they taste better and are more fulfilling than processed foods.

Question: I have diabetes (or cancer, heart disease, etc), what is the best plan of action for me?

Answer: Of course you should consult with your doctor to address your specific medical situation, especially if you are taking blood thinners or other types of medication. In general an exclusively whole food diet will allow your body to halt and even reverse most preventable diseases. Adopt a balanced whole food diet, get plenty of exercise and ample sleep, your body will do the rest. Avoid the trap of self medicating with supplements or chasing other quick fixes. There are no magic bullets. Your body is designed for a whole food diet, just give your body what it needs.

2 - Why The American Diet is Killing Us

I wish it would be as easy as just saying processed food and factory farmed animal products are bad, and leave it at that. If that were the case we could start with the fun stuff, like shopping for food and cooking. However, processed food is addictive and it's everywhere. Rejecting processed food will not be easy, so it's important to have a good understanding of the underlying issues.

The modern American diet is built on a foundation of processed food and factory farmed animal products. It is called the modern American diet because it originated in the United States and is the brainchild of the American food industry. The modern American diet has spread to most other countries, American fast food and processed food is available worldwide. Not wanting to miss out on a lucrative opportunity, food industries in other countries now sell similar products.

The American food industry is proud of their accomplishments. One of the things the food industry regards as a major accomplishment is the reduction of food costs as a percentage of total household spending, due to advances in factory farming and food processing. This was accomplished while increasing profits to the industry. The industry is also proud of advances in processing and preservatives that have increased the shelf life of food, helping to reduce spoilage and further increase profits. While at first this may sound like a win-win situation for both the food industry and for consumers, it clearly is not. The only winner is the food industry, consumers are the losers.

The modern American diet causes millions of deaths each year from preventable disease such as cancer, cardiovascular and heart disease, diabetes, Alzheimer's, autoimmune problems and obesity. More than 90% of of the American population over 50 is on medication. Over 33% of Americans are obese and over 70% are overweight. Even with modern medical advances, the life expectancy in the United States is going down, because of the American diet. This means that your children may die before you do.

Not only is the American diet killing people, but it is destroying our quality of life and the economy. Living on medication for years with serious illness is not a good way to live. Fighting to maintain dignity and self esteem because of obesity is no way to live. The huge medical bills and outrageous insurance rates caused by the American diet puts stress on everyone and destroys the economy while the food and medical industries make record profits.

The wrong fuel

A quick analogy; Most cars are made to run on gasoline. Did you ever wonder what would happen if you put pure alcohol in the gas tank of your car? Or oil? A good guess is that bad things will happen. For this reason you only put gas in your car. You don't try other types of fuel, because gas is the fuel that your car is designed to use. The human body is also designed for a specific type of fuel. The human body is designed for whole food. Since the first human beings walked the earth, we have eaten a diet of whole food. With a whole food diet humans do not suffer from high rates of obesity and preventable diseases.

About 70 years ago our diet changed with the increasing use of processed foods and factory farmed animal products. With this new diet came obesity and disease. Why? Because processed foods and factory farmed animal products are the wrong fuel for our bodies. They are not what your body is designed for. The interactions between our metabolic systems and food are complex and there are many factors that contribute to the poor performance of the modern American diet, but they all stem from the same basic issue, the modern American diet is the wrong fuel for the human body, just as pancake syrup is the wrong fuel for your car.

How processed foods became so prevalent

Before we get into the details of how processed foods are made and exactly what they do to your body, lets see when and why they came into such widespread use. During World War 2 (1939-1945) the United States supplied food to millions of troops worldwide. The food industry was asked to develop processed foods with improved preservatives to prevent the food from going bad during shipment and storage. Huge factories were built to make processed food. The long term health effects of processed food were not studied, the focus was on the short term goal of producing large quantities of food as efficiently as possible to support the war.

At the war's end the United States faced a possible economic crisis if they shut down factories that were built to supply the war effort. To keep factories running they needed a new market. They decided to develop the consumer market. During the war there was a culture of frugality. Everything was rationed and people were encouraged to consume as little as possible. After the war both business and government wanted to create a consumer culture and to promote consumption to maintain a strong economy. To cause this change, powerful advertising was used to promote the idea that consuming is good and that it is fun to be a consumer. It took several years of intensive promotion, but by the 1950's development of the consumer culture was well under way.

By the time the consumer culture was taking off, the American food industry realized that selling processed food was far more profitable than selling whole food, so they made selling processed food their top priority. Over the next 60 years the market share for processed food steadily increased. Today most of the food in an American grocery store consists of processed food or factory farmed animal products. The US government assisted the food industry in developing and promoting these products, but did little to study the long term health implications. Instead of protecting the people, the US government mislead the people with guidelines like the USDA food pyramid that promoted consumption of processed foods and factory farmed animal products.

To add a visual perspective to when the modern American diet became mainstream, we can look at pictures from the last 100 years. One collection of pictures shows people in swimsuits from 1900 to 2000. From 1900 to 1950 most people in the US look fit and healthy. Beginning in the 1950's the level of fitness starts to decline each year. By the year 2000 a disturbingly high percentage of people are overweight and even obese. This timeline coincides with the rise of the consumer culture and the increased use of processed food and factory farmed animal products. Processed food and factory farmed animal products are now the cornerstone of the American diet and are spreading to most other countries around the world.

How processed foods are made

Most processed food is made from whole food which is changed in some way (processed). Whole food is raw and unbroken food as it came from the plant. The processing of food can take many forms but usually includes the following steps:

1. The outer covering of the plant is removed such as the shell, hull, bran or skin.
2. The innermost part of the plant is removed (if there is one). This includes seeds, pit, germ or core.
3. What remains is pulverized or ground, resulting in juice, paste or dry particles.
4. The juice, paste or dry particles are strained or filtered.
5. Further refinement is done. Refinement means that different constituents (original parts) are separated or removed and additional grinding is done to reduce the size of the particles. In addition to grinding, chemicals are sometimes used including acids and bleaches. After refinement most processed foods have a higher energy density. This means that they have higher calories but less nutrients.
6. Modification and treatment is done using substances and chemicals to achieve the desired consistency, taste and shelf life of the finished product. These substances can include acidity regulators, anti-caking agents, anti-foaming agents, antioxidants, bulking agents, food coloring, color retention agents, emulsifiers, flavors, flavor enhancers, flour treatment agents, glazing agents, humectants, tracer gases, preservatives, stabilizers, sweeteners and thickeners. Some of the chemicals used to treat food are carcinogenic (known to cause cancer).
7. Some processing stages are done at high temperatures that kill nutritional value and cause the formation of acrylamide, furan and other cancer forming substances.

8. In some cases several processed ingredients are combined and then heated or baked to create a finished product (such as bread, crackers, cookies, chips, snack food, etc).

Processed foods cause weight gain

Your digestive system is designed to do all of the digestion (refining) that your body needs. Processed foods are already refined so that when you eat processed food you are eating the equivalent of pre-digested food. Processed food has a higher energy density level (too much energy) and your body was not designed for this.

When you eat processed foods your body puts refined sugars into your bloodstream almost immediately. Once this energy is in your bloodstream your body must reduce your blood sugar to a safe level or you will become sick. There are only three ways that your body can reduce your blood sugar level:

1. Convert the sugar to fat and store the fat on your body. This is what normally happens. To do this your body produces insulin to trigger the conversion of unwanted sugar into fat. This is why eating processed food causes such rapid weight gain.

2. Burn the sugar by raising your body temperature. This is called thermal dissipation. This is what your body does when you have a fever or to keep you warm in cold weather. Thermal dissipation is not a practical option for reducing blood sugar levels because it would take too long. You could take off all your clothes and jump into freezing water to force your body to burn some of this energy, but only a crazy person would do this.

3. Burn the sugar using your muscles by doing some type of vigorous exercise. This is a bad option, because it would take a tremendous amount of exercise to prevent your body from doing option #1 (converting the sugar to fat). Only a crazy person would run a marathon every day, just to eat processed food without gaining weight.

The sensible solution is to eat whole foods. When you eat whole foods it takes hours for your body to digest them. This gives you a slow release of energy as you need it, and does not spike your insulin levels to cause your fat storage mode to kick in. This is the reason why whole food keeps you from getting hungry for so much longer than processed foods.

Hey! the gas gauge is broken

When you eat processed foods your body can't tell when you have eaten enough, it thinks you are always hungry. This makes you overeat. When eating processed food, if you don't want to overeat you must stop eating while you are still hungry. This takes a lot of discipline and is not fun. On the other hand, with a diet of whole foods your gas gauge works properly and you don't need to worry about overeating or walking around hungry. If you are really hungry you can eat a huge plate of lower calorie whole foods and literally stuff yourself with no concerns! This is totally guilt free and you feel great later.

Processed foods are stripped of nutritional value

In steps 1 through 5 of food processing (from the list earlier in this chapter) the nutritive parts of the plant are removed and discarded. What is left is further refined, often at high temperatures and using harsh chemicals. This strips most or all of the nutritional value from the food. In a feeble attempt to restore some of the lost nutritional value, vitamins and minerals are sometimes added to the finished products. However, these are often chemical versions of vitamins and not in the best form for use by the human body. Adding vitamins to compensate for nutritionally deficient processed foods is known as fortification. Common processed foods with fortification are fortified milk, fortified orange juice and fortified breakfast cereal. Fortification can't replace the wide spectrum of nutrients that are in whole foods.

You can't believe what's on the label

When was the last time you heard of a food supplier receiving a penalty for having a discrepancy about the ingredients listed (or not listed) on a food label? If you research this, you will find that when a labeling discrepancy is discovered, it is not a very serious issue unless someone was poisoned or otherwise sickened and there was gross negligence proven in a court of law. Many ingredients such as emulsifiers, solvents and some preservatives fall into the category of "incidental ingredients" and are not even required to be listed on food labels! Furthermore there is no requirement to list the toxins that are in processed foods. The reasoning given for this is that a toxin is not an intended ingredient. Nevertheless, if suppliers know that there are toxins such as mercury and BPA in foods, why shouldn't the supplier have a duty to inform the consumer of this? Until now the technology to test food to determine the actual ingredients has been very expensive, so widespread testing is not done. Hopefully this will change and bring a greater level of honesty to the food industry. This is one more reason to avoid processed food. With processed food you don't really know what you are eating.

Processed food promotes cancer and disease

Processed food promotes cancer and disease in many ways. Every ounce of nutritionally deficient processed food you eat is an ounce of nutritional whole food you will not eat. Because your body was designed for 100% whole foods, this loss of nutritional value will cause you to have nutritional deficiencies and a loss of immunity to diseases. This explains why malnutrition often accompanies obesity with a diet that is high in processed foods. This loss of nutrients can not be restored by taking vitamins and supplements.

The reason why vitamins and supplements cannot restore the nutritional value is that they are incomplete and provide only a small fraction of the nutrients that are present in whole foods.

Processed foods with high energy densities (refined sugars) promote cancer and heart disease. Think of high energy processed foods as cancer food. Do you really want to feed cancer? Not only that, but high energy density food increases your metabolism which increases aging. Do you really want to get old faster? Last but not least, most processed foods contain cancer causing chemicals and substances. Some of these are inter-process chemicals that are not even listed on food labels.

Factory farmed animal products are processed foods

Factory farmed animal products are a processed food. This is because factory farmed animals eat a diet consisting of mostly processed fodder (animal food). Processed fodder has all of the same problems that processed foods for humans have, along with a few more serious problems. Fodder is usually lower quality than processed food for humans and has more contaminants. You may be wondering why it matters what the animals eat, after all we won't be eating their food. It matters because many of the toxins that the animals eat, such as mercury, arsenic, PCB's, pesticides, fungicides and antibiotics are trapped in the animals body and end up in the products we eat.

It gets worse. Not only are toxins trapped in the animals body, but some toxins are magnified. This is known as biomagnification. This is a fancy way of saying that some of the toxins the animal eats over its entire lifetime are stored in the fatty tissues of that animal. When you eat the animal you get that animals entire lifetime accumulation of toxins. By eating meat your dose of toxins is much higher than if you ate plant based foods. This is a good reason to reduce or eliminate meat from your diet.

Dairy problems

Dairy includes milk, cheese, butter, ice cream and yogurt. In addition many of the ingredients used in processed foods are made from dairy. Most dairy is made from cows milk. Cows' milk is made by mother cows' for a specific purpose, to cause rapid cell growth and weight gain in baby cows'. Cows' milk causes rapid cell growth and weight gain in humans as well, including cancer cells. Our bodies were not designed for dairy. Cows' milk is designed to take a baby cow from 100 pounds to over 1000 pounds in less than a year! Cows' milk contains high levels of IGF-1 (insulin-like growth factor 1) which causes rapid aging and promotes the growth of many types of cancers.

Animal protein from dairy and meat causes calcium loss and osteoporosis. This is counter intuitive so I will repeat it again; animal based foods including dairy cause osteoporosis and bone density loss! This is because as your body processes animal protein it produces acid. Your body uses calcium from your bones to reduce the level of this acid. Although dairy has calcium in it, the amount of calcium that is used to process animal protein is greater than the amount of calcium that can be assimilated from the dairy. This is known as net calcium depletion. The USDA sure isn't telling us this! This is why countries with the highest consumption of animal protein have the greatest number of people with osteoporosis.

Dairy is high in saturated fat that causes heart disease. Low fat or fat free dairy is not the answer because it contains even higher levels of IGF-1 (Insulin-like growth factor 1) which promotes cancer. Factory farmed dairy can contain antibiotics, hormones and fungicides, that are used to maximize production.

Norway historically has high levels of dairy and meat consumption and high levels of heart disease. During WW2 Germany took over Norway and absconded with all dairy and meat for their own use. This resulted in a huge reduction of heart disease in Norway during the war. After the war heart disease quickly returned to the pre-war levels with the reintroduction of dairy and meat. Tests with laboratory animals produce the same results; with high consumption of dairy the disease levels increase, when dairy is removed the disease levels rapidly decrease.

Factory farmed meat problems

All meat contains animal protein, even lean meat and white meat. Animal protein is directly linked to many forms of cancer and to heart disease. The greater the quantity consumed, the stronger the link to these diseases.

Saturated animal fat is contained in all meat, lean meat has less, but still has a lot. Factory farmed meat that is labeled as lean is only lean when compared to regular factory farmed meat, it is not actually lean. No factory farmed meat qualifies as being lean when compared to the wild animals that were eaten by humans historically. Saturated animal fat lines the walls of arteries with plaque and causes cardiovascular disease, strokes and blood clots.

Some factory farmed meat contains bovine growth hormones that are used to make the animals grow faster. These hormones cause the animal to grow differently than an undrugged animal and causes the meat to have less nutritional value. When you eat the meat, you are also eating some amount of the growth hormones.

Antibiotics and fungicides are routinely used in a prophylactic mode to enable factory farmed animals to survive under horrible conditions. This means that they are administered to many or all animals, not just those that are sick.

Factory farming of animals has huge environmental impacts. Meat production uses ten times more fuel than plant based products. The grain that is used for factory farmed animals could feed over a billion people that now go hungry in poor countries. Factory farming of animals uses large amounts of water leading to water shortages. Factory farming is cruel and inhumane to the animals. The poor conditions and overcrowding of animals can lead to the rapid incubation, mutation and spread of diseases that cause human pandemics like swine flu and bird flu.

Factory farmed vegetable problems

Factory farming is another name for large scale industrial farming. It is also called intensive farming. The main problem with the factory farming of vegetables and staple crops is that profits are a higher priority than long term health. This manifests itself in every decision made by factory farms including the following:

- Heavy use of chemical fertilizers and pesticides to maximize crop yield.
- Widespread use of human waste (biosolids) as a fertilizer!
- Crops are selected and bred for quantity instead of nutritional value.
- Monocrops cause lack of diversity in the food supply system.
- Genetically modified organisms are often used.

Human waste (sewage sludge from sewage treatment plants) is used as a fertilizer in many factory farms. It is called **biosolids** to make it sound better. Although recycling is good in theory, using sewage sludge from municipal treatment plants to fertilize food crops is a bad idea. The problem is that sewage sludge contains toxic heavy metals and pollutants such as mercury, lead, arsenic, cadmium, barium, chromium, manganese, steroids, hormones, endocrine disruptors, PCB's, dioxin, brominated flame retardants and human pathogens such as staphylococcus aureus. This is just a partial list. These toxins cannot be properly filtered or removed from biosolids and accumulate in the soil.

One of the biggest problems with the use of sewage sludge is that it is used on feed crops for factory farmed animals as well. Because of the biomagnification that we talked about earlier in the chapter, the animals act as chemical concentrators and accumulate the toxins in their bodies. When we eat factory farmed animal products we are getting an amped-up (amplified) dose of these toxins.

Before 1992 most cities dumped their sewage sludge into the ocean. The US government banned ocean dumping in 1992 and many other counties enacted similar bans to save the oceans. They needed a new way to get rid of the sludge. Landfills were expensive, so they came up with the not-so-bright idea of using the sludge as fertilizer for farms. They are getting away with this because it takes years for the effects of the poisoning to be seen and by the time it is, it is hard to pin down a single instance or location. Factory farmers will say that it is not their products that caused the problem, it is some other source. Proving which source caused health problems years later is difficult or impossible.

An example of a monocrop is the modern corn you see in most grocery stores. This corn is bred for large size and high growth rates at the expense of good taste and nutritional value. On many farms this is the only thing planted, hence the "mono" in monocrop which means one. The problem with one crop instead of rotating multiple types of crops is that the soil requires greater amounts of chemical fertilizers. Furthermore, insect pests become adapted to the monocrop and require ever increasing amounts of pesticides to be used. Monocrop soil has less minerals and nutrients. This is important because trace amounts of soil get into the food and this is a vital source of minerals and nutrients to the people that eat the food.

The reductionist approach

The reductionist approach is the approach used by the American food industry. The reductionist approach focuses on individual substances and foods and the profits they can generate, instead of the nutritional benefits of the entire diet. This produces disastrous results because it ignores the complex interactions between nutrients and the body's systems, and disregards most long term health consequences. The big picture approach is the opposite of the reductionist approach and focuses on the overall health impact of food products and how they fit into the overall diet.

There should be a balance between profit and long term health consequences, but when millions of people are dying from preventable diseases in a scientifically advanced society, it's clear that big picture issues are not being addressed. If you are interested in reading more about this, a good book on the subject is "Whole" by T. Colin Campbell. This book talks about why important research findings in the area of nutrition are ignored by the food industry and our society. Dr. Campbell is one of the top nutritional research scientists in the world and has done highly acclaimed peer-reviewed research, such as spearheading the China-Cornell-Oxford project.

Why doesn't the government protect us?

What about the USDA and FDA? Unfortunately these agencies do little to protect us in terms of long term health, because they are indirectly being controlled by the food industry. There is a revolving door policy and top decision makers freely rotate positions between these agencies and leading food manufacturers. The only way to put a stop to this is to change the laws that govern how these agencies are run, but with the present corporate control of the political system the situation is unlikely to change anytime soon.

Frequently Asked Questions

Question: You appear to be negative towards corporations, the government and the food industry, what is your position?

Answer: My position is that health and well being has taken a back seat to profit and it's gone too far. People should come first. Many people should not lose their health and even their life so that a few people can make huge profits. The present situation is out of control and is not in the best interest of the people or the country. Our country is transforming from a proud and powerful country to the land of sickness and obesity.

Question: How do you know if a food is a processed food?

Answer: Many types of processed foods are made to look like natural food, so it can be difficult to tell which foods are processed. There is no standard labeling for disclosing which foods are processed and what type of processing has been done to them. Having terms like "natural", "whole" and "organic" printed on the packaging tells you little or nothing. For this reason you should assume that all foods are processed unless you are sure that they are not.

Most food served in restaurants is processed or made from factory farmed animal products. There are no labels on restaurant food, so you don't know what the ingredients are. For the most part restaurant food tends to be the worst food you can get with large amounts of fat, sugar and salt. For this reason I rarely eat at restaurants, and watch very closely what I am eating if I do. If you need to eat at restaurants there are some strategies to help minimize the damage. We will talk about these in chapter three.

Question: how much processed food, dairy or factory farmed animal products can I eat without compromising my health or causing weight gain?

Answer: Personally I try to limit it to under 1 or 2 percent of my total calories. Ask yourself what percentage of health problems are you willing to tolerate. Since you normally have little indication that health problems are mounting, it is best to be on the safe side. Since bad food feeds cancer and heart disease ask yourself how much cancer and heart disease are you willing to tolerate? Another consideration is the simplicity of a whole food diet. As we will discuss in chapter four, a whole food diet supplies all of your nutritional requirements with very few additional concerns. The more you deviate from a straight whole food diet the more complicated your diet will become.

3 - Making The Change

It seems like it should be easy. Stop eating harmful foods and replace them with whole foods. For this you will have a longer and healthier life with a major reduction or complete elimination of most diseases. So why are most people still allowing a bad diet to destroy their health?

One reason is that to get the total benefit of a whole food diet requires a complete rejection of the American diet including processed food and factory farmed animal products. This necessitates a serious commitment and strong willpower. Most people underestimate the difficulty and fall short of meeting the challenge. Think of it as if you are going to war and you will be fighting for your life, because actually that's what it is. As in war you must do everything that is needed to come out on top. Ruthlessly crush food addictions, social pressure, old habits and anything else that stands in your way. With this type of determination will you succeed.

There is no one-size-fits-all approach to changing your diet. Personalities vary greatly, what works for one person may not work for another. Some people are able to throw the switch and never look back, for others it is much more difficult. You will need to design a customized game plan that will work for you. Be honest with yourself about your strengths and weaknesses and plan accordingly. The rest of this chapter presents ideas that can be used to design your own personalized battle plan. Think of it as a toolbox. Select the ideas that will work best for you. Most importantly find that switch, that point at which you know what needs to be done and will let nothing stop you!

If you are trying to lose weight

To lose weight permanently, you must remove all processed food from your diet. Processed food = fat food, it's that simple. It takes surprisingly little processed food to sabotage your attempts at weight loss. Depending on your metabolism, it can take as little as a few pieces of processed bread here and some processed salad dressing there and you will have no progress. Once you lose weight you must continue to stay off the processed food or you will gain the weight back again. It's a choice you have to make; processed food and weight gain or whole foods and a natural trim weight. You can't have both, its one or the other.

If you are young and have a high metabolism you may be able to get away with eating processed foods for a while, but it won't last. After a few years you will gain weight. Instead, you should change your diet now, before you experience the weight gain and health issues that come with the American diet.

Food addictions

You're addicted! We are all programmed from birth with a mild to medium addiction to sugar, fat and salt. If we eat foods that are high in sugar, fat and salt, this addiction becomes stronger. We are programmed this way for a reason. The human body was designed for food scarcity.

The human body was designed to acquire and store energy. Our ancestors often had no idea when their next meal would come. They needed to travel long distances and go for days at a time without food if necessary. To make this possible the human brain is programmed to crave high energy food and the body is programmed to store the energy from this food. This causes us to eat large amounts of food when it is available. Our body stores the energy as fat, so that it can power our body later when we need it.

While this programming served us well in the past, it causes problems in the modern day world of processed food. Our programming is not calibrated for high energy processed food. A modern sedentary lifestyle with low physical activity compounds the problem. The only permanent solution is to remove processed food from our diet.

There is no way to change your programming and force your body to function correctly with processed foods. Some companies advertise fad products and drugs that they claim will reprogram the metabolic system, but this is a deception to take your money. Either these products do not work or they contain dangerous drugs such as amphetamines that will raise your metabolism by increasing your heart rate, even while at rest. None of these products result in a permanent change and many have been taken off the market, because they cause heart failure or other complications.

The food industry creates products that cause food addictions. If you don't believe it, try to change your diet and you will quickly understand how powerful these addictions are. Some researchers think that food addictions are harder to break than smoking, alcohol or drug addictions.

Do not underestimate how difficult it is to stop eating processed foods and to eliminate factory farmed animal products from your diet. You will be fighting a psychological battle and your internal programming will be acting against you. I say this not to be discouraging, but because if you have a realistic picture of what you are up against, it will improve your chances for success.

Many people rationalize their failure to change diets and convince themselves that it is just a minor problem to be solved another day, no big deal. They do this for years and claim that they are really not addicted and that they can stop eating processed foods any time they want to, they are just not ready yet! The best approach is to recognize how serious this problem is and to take the needed steps to defeat it. Sometimes drastic steps are needed, but ultimately these additions can be broken.

Eating whole foods may seem strange

Most people say that it feels strange to eat different foods than they are used to eating. They feel like they are missing something and have a strong urge to go back to their old ways of eating. This is because any way of eating is habit forming and there are strong behavioral forces that try to keep us doing the same thing we are used to. This is normal, and it will subside after a while as your new diet becomes a habit and replaces your old diet. If you have perseverance you can make the change.

Social perspective

There are complex social aspects surrounding diet and food selection. This explains the extreme polarization some people exhibit in regard to diets and nutrition. Throughout history, diet and food selection have played a role in social grouping. Diet and food selection are often used as a display of common values or to show loyalty in relationships. Changing eating habits can be perceived as weakening these relationships or even as a betrayal.

In modern society we have better ways to establish social grouping than through food. We no longer need to use food to display our common values or to show loyalty. We should choose our food and diet solely on the basis of what is best for our long term health. Unfortunately these behavioral and social aspects of diet and food selection are still very much alive in the modern world and touch everyone to some degree. Do what is right for your health and make rational and fact based decisions about your diet and food selection.

Internal Programming

When you think of social pressure, external pressure from family and peers probably comes to mind, however the most powerful pressure comes from inside us. We are internally hard wired to conform to social norms. Most of us reject the suggestion that the pressure to conform can affect our choices. We like to believe that we are independent thinkers. For this reason we recite a broad assortment of excuses to explain why we are unable to change our eating habits.

Going against social norms makes us an outsider. This makes most people uncomfortable and in some cases can feel downright bad. Most people will go to great lengths to avoid being the outsider. When over seventy percent of the food in the average grocery store is either processed food or factory farmed animal products you are a social outsider when you eliminate these foods from your diet. Even worse is that almost all of the foods that are advertised on television are processed foods or factory farmed animal products.

Eating a whole food diet puts you directly at odds with your internal bias to conform to social norms. This can be difficult to overcome, particularly if you do not understand where the pressure is coming from. Once aware, some people are able to overcome this by sheer willpower alone. Most people will have to take additional measures. If you are able to associate yourself with other like minded people you will be an insider in this smaller group and can support each other. This will give you a tremendous psychological advantage.

Strategies

Cold Turkey

In this strategy you immediately and completely change your diet with no transition period. This may be difficult if you have limited experience cooking and preparing whole foods. It takes some time to learn to cook and prepare whole foods, there is some trial and error that you will go through. If you want to make the change cold turkey, you may want to spend a few weeks cooking and preparing whole foods, then make the change. This way you will have found meals that you like and will be comfortable with them.

A big advantage of going cold turkey is that you can clean out your entire kitchen to remove the foods you no longer want. Not having to see these foods every time you walk into the kitchen will reduce your temptation. During the transition period you are more vulnerable while you are retraining your taste perceptions and fighting food addictions.

Making the transition immediately (cold turkey) is much more likely to succeed than any other method. Think about what it would be like for an alcoholic to stop drinking by reducing consumption little by little each day. Vodka is in the living room, wine is in the kitchen and beer in the game room. Sounds unlikely to succeed doesn't it? On the other hand if all alcohol is removed and the change is immediate, the chance of success is much greater.

Slow Transition

In this strategy you change your diet gradually over a period of time. People with family members who are resistant to change may find this strategy attractive. The down side of a slow transition is that food from your old diet is still in the house. This makes it more difficult to avoid temptation. One idea is to do it in steps. Remove major offenders like refined sugar or processed foods first. A while later you can go to the next step and eliminate factory farmed animal products. Keep in mind that a slow transition is much less likely to be successful.

Substitution

In this strategy offending foods are replaced with healthy alternatives. This can work one of two ways:

- Use healthy recipes to replace the unhealthy food and processed foods in your diet. You will prepare the healthy recipes yourself, so that you have control over the ingredients and how the food is prepared. This can be an effective solution.

- Buy "health food" to replace regular processed food. Many people try this unsuccessfully. It is a bad idea and does not work because most health food is really not healthy, it is just a slightly better version of processed food.

Avoid this mistake

When transitioning to a whole food diet, it is a mistake to immediately start eating a lot of raw vegetables. It takes time to build up the beneficial bacteria in your system that will allow you to efficiently digest raw vegetables. Many people who start with a lot of raw vegetables upset their digestive system. When this happens they assume that "a whole food diet is not compatible with my digestive system". This is not true. Everyone's digestive system is basically the same, however it may take a few weeks to a couple months to develop the bacteria needed to digest raw vegetables properly.

Lightly cooking your vegetables will kill bacteria that is unfriendly to your digestive system. Gradually start eating raw vegetables. If you find that your digestive system is getting upset, back off for a few days until your system recovers.

You may experience withdrawal symptoms

Processed foods and factory farmed animal products are addictive, so you may experience withdrawal symptoms. During withdrawal your brain makes you have cravings or feel bad, in an attempt to force you to resume eating the addictive food. DONT GIVE IN! In terms of brain function, this is the same as going through withdrawal from drugs.

Reprogramming your mind and your taste

Keep in mind that processed food manufacturers have "flavorists" and "taste engineers" that have turned seasoning into a science and use artificial chemicals to flavor foods. These taste engineers have basically unlimited time and budgets to make ever more intense and captivating flavors. Seasonings for whole foods can't compete with artificial flavorings as far as delivering an addictively intense "flavor burst" every time you take a bite of food.

For this reason you should give your taste buds a chance to re-calibrate if you are making the transition from a standard American diet. For the first couple months a whole food diet may taste bland. After your taste buds adjust you will find that natural seasonings actually taste better than the artificial ones used in processed foods. You will also taste the foods themselves. Unlike processed foods that are flavorless and must be heavily seasoned to make a finished product, whole foods have a great natural taste to them and do not require heavy seasoning.

- The better your new food tastes the higher your chance of success! Take the time to learn to cook and season whole foods and you will increase your chance of success.
- Cut down on meat by eating small portions and eating it very slowly so that the length of time you are eating is the same as before, but the quantity is much less.
- Use meat as a side dish or use small pieces to spice up vegetable based dishes.
- If you like to "enjoy your food" there will be a time period of a few months before your taste will re-calibrate and you will start enjoying your new diet.

Avoiding temptation

In the list below are some ideas for avoiding temptation. If you find that you are succumbing to temptation and these items don't help, do some soul searching as to why, then devise your own way to stay on track.

- Figure out what foods you like. Cook a supply in advance and store it in sealable containers, so you always have something healthy to eat that is readily available.
- Keep a supply of healthy food you can munch on, such as fruits, veggies or trail mix. This will keep you from getting hungry and going off-diet.
- Don't get caught off guard. When someone offers you food that is off-diet, respond firmly and without hesitation. Maintain your willpower.
- Remove all food that is off-diet from your kitchen.
- Talk to family and friends, try to get them to cooperate and not eat off-diet foods around you if possible.
- Avoid most restaurants. See the section below "Restaurants and Restaurant Food".
- Make a deal with yourself - If you eat something off diet, you must exercise and work off the same amount of calories immediately. This is a way of acknowledging what you are eating and will cause you to eat less of the offending foods.
- Reward yourself - Take a vacation if you have stayed on track for some period of time.

Creating your support system

Use the buddy system for support if possible. You may be able to find a buddy to change your diet with, because most people want to make a change.

People in your household can be one of your biggest challenges, if they are bringing processed food and factory farmed animal products into your house. Seeing processed food in your kitchen many times a day can undermine your resolve. Encourage them to support your new diet. Children should be a part of your support system. See the section below "Making The Change With Children".

There are a number of twelve step programs available for food addictions that are based on the twelve step AA (Alcoholics anonymous) program. These programs are supposed to create a support system with other people that have similar goals. On the surface this seems like a good idea, but for some reason the success rate for twelve step programs is low. However, if this type of program can work for you, then why not?

Restaurants and restaurant food

It is hard to give up the shared social experience of eating together, but most restaurant food is detrimental, because it's high in saturated fat, sugar and salt. There is no transparency and no list of the ingredients at most restaurants. The reason why restaurant food is high in fat, sugar and salt is to addict you and keep you coming back. Fast food is usually the worst, but regular restaurants can be very bad as well. The best defense against restaurant food is to not eat at restaurants! This approach will save a lot of money.

Many types of food served in restaurants such as salad and fruit are sprayed with chemicals to prevent them from turning brown or rotting. This allows the salad to appear fresh for many hours but these chemicals are bad for your health and can make you sick or cause digestive problems such as bowel irritation and diarrhea. This is not such a big problem for people who eat small amounts of salad, but for people who eat large salads this is a serious problem.

Some ideas for when you do eat at a restaurant:

- Try to eat at restaurants that will customize your order. You can specify dishes like steamed vegetables.

- Do not use processed salad dressings. Even low fat dressings are sometimes not really low in fat or have other undesirable ingredients in place of the fat.

- Avoid food with oil because oil is a processed food and is very high in calories. Olive oil or canola oil may be better choices than lard, but they are still processed foods that cause weight gain.

- Try to eat small amounts.

If you often eat at restaurants in a social or business setting, you may come to the point where you have to put your health first. This can be a tough decision, because many people are convinced that forgoing restaurants would make networking difficult. Don't let the combination of business or social activities sabotage your health.

Making the change with children

Children learn most things from their peer group. If you want to change a child's eating habits, you should take their peer group into account. Using the direct approach of mandating a change against their peer group is unlikely to be successful. Children are extremely susceptible to advertising, that's why so much money is spent on advertising to children. The characters in advertising become an extension of the child's peer group. It is your job to protect them from this powerful threat.

Most school lunches are shamefully bad and consist mostly of low quality processed foods and factory farmed animal products. My suggestion is to prepare your child's lunches at home.

Fasting to break stubborn food addictions

If you are having a difficult time breaking food addictions and changing your diet, you could try fasting. Fasting is a way of doing a system reset to break food addictions. Food addictions are like a bad software routine that is installed in your brain. Fasting can be used to uninstall the bad routine. Fasting is also a mechanism your body uses to repair itself. One reason that you lose your appetite when you are sick is that your body is causing you to fast. This slows down many of your bodies systems and gives your body a chance to repair itself. See your doctor before you try fasting to make sure that you will not have medical complications and that it is safe for you to fast.

Sometimes fasting may not be possible, for example in situations where you need to perform with a clear mind and make important decisions that affect safety, such as driving a motor vehicle. This is because fasting can make you feel dizzy and nauseous. In this case you may be able to get most of the benefit of fasting by near-fasting. This is usually done by eating a low calorie food such as cabbage. This allows you to fill your stomach, but still has low enough energy to cause your body to go into a fasting mode. Near-fasting is much more comfortable than a full fast. For more information about fasting, a book that covers breaking food addictions and fasting is "The Pleasure Trap" by Douglas J. Lisle, PH.D.

If at first you don't succeed, try try try again

If you don't succeed, then regroup and reflect on what went wrong. Make changes to your game plan and try again. Some people require several attempts, with each attempt working better than the last. DO NOT GET DISCOURAGED! Remember, this is serious business. Don't give up. Keep attacking the problem from different angles until you prevail. You can do this. Your health and your life depend on it.

Overcoming self destructive behavior

Self destructive behavior can be a big problem. If you can't make sense of your eating habits, your eating habits may have little to do with food and could be caused by self destructive behavior. It is important to untangle the motivational factors that drive your eating habits. If you find that you are engaging in self destructive behavior, take steps to identify and address the underlying causes.

Tips and ideas

Pray - If you are religious you can pray for the strength to overcome food addictions and make the change of diet. The Bible talks of not debasing your body, the modern American diet is certainly debasing the body! If you believe in the marvel of the human body, you should respect your body and its intended food source, which is NOT the modern American diet.

Temporarily relocate - As a last resort, temporarily relocate. If your home environment, family or associations are making it impossible to change your diet, you may need to leave for a while so that you can make the change. If you know people that eat correctly and will help you, then perhaps you can stay with them for a while until you have adjusted to your new diet. There are also programs that are set up for this purpose. Some of these programs combine diet and exercise routines.

4 - Nutritional Foundation for Optimum Health

The most reliable way to determine if a diet is healthy or unhealthy is through large scale scientific studies and health data. Large scale scientific studies and health data were used to prove that smoking causes cancer, something that the tobacco companies denied for years. Because large scale scientific studies and health data involve many people, they are reliable and it is difficult for special interests (like the food industry) to skew the results.

What the data tells us

A whole food diet with minimal amounts of processed food and animal products results in superior health and a large reduction in preventable diseases. Some diseases can be nearly eliminated. The following data makes this clear:

- The EPIC study in Europe is a study of 500,000 people in 23 countries. The EPIC study shows that increased consumption of vegetables and fruits lowers most forms of preventable disease and increases life expectancy. EPIC also shows that high blood sugar levels associated with processed foods promote cardiovascular disease and that consumption of processed meat is associated with cardiovascular disease and cancer.

- The China-Cornell-Oxford Project (China Study) is a study of 6500 people in China. The China Study shows that a plant based diet is the healthiest diet and that consumption of animal protein is associated with cancer and cardiovascular disease.

- World Health Organization country-by-country data shows that people in countries with higher consumption of processed foods have higher rates of heart disease and cancer. Countries with higher consumption of dairy products suffer from higher instances of cancer and osteoporosis.

- World Health Organization mortality data shows that affluent countries with a diet high in processed foods and factory farmed animal products have higher mortality rates from cardiovascular disease, cancer, diabetes and Alzheimer's disease.

In chapter twelve the web sites for these studies are listed. You can read the findings and in some cases the entire data sets can be downloaded if you want to review the data yourself.

What history says

To find the optimum diet, we should look back on our long term history to see what we ate before industrialization. This idea should not be confused with the recently popular paleo diet. The paleo diet starts out along the same lines, but is based on the incorrect assumption that humans had a historical diet without grains or legumes and with large amounts of meat. It should be noted however, that the paleo diet rightly rejects processed foods, dairy and factory farmed animal products.

Modern research shows that the historical human diet varied according to time and geographic location. While some small northern populations in cold climates had higher meat consumption (and shorter life expectancies), the vast majority of humans had a whole food diet with low to moderate meat consumption. The meat was very lean and free of contaminants. Part of the meat was in the form of insects and eggs. Our historical diet included grains and legumes, although not the modern varieties that are a result of selective breeding.

On the subject of selective breeding, it is notable that most modern food is a result of selective breeding, and is substantially different than the original species. This includes most vegetables, fruits, nuts, grains, berries, seeds, legumes, tubers, animals, even some fish. Fortunately, with only a few exceptions the selectively bred versions we have now are not nutritionally deficient and can provide the basis for a healthy whole food diet.

Historically there was no dairy in the human diet before the domestication of farm animals. There was no processed food or factory farmed animal products in the human diet. Our digestive system and anatomy have not recently changed and we have not substantially adapted to dairy, processed foods or factory farmed animal products. Our diet throughout 99% of the history of our species, has been a whole food diet with low to moderate consumption of lean meat, eggs and insects.

The optimum diet

The optimum diet presented in this book is based on our historical whole food diet. The large scale studies and world health organization data confirm this to be the best diet for long term health.

Although based on our historical diet, this is not an exact recreation of the historical human diet. There are some notable differences and adaptations. Modern varieties of whole foods are used, because that is what is now available. Consumption of meat and animal products is reduced. Ancient people had a limited life expectancy, so the disease causing aspects of eating meat and animal products was not a concern (and was unknown at the time). In addition, the lean meat that was eaten historically was of far better quality than the meat that is readily available to us now.

With a whole food diet your body will regulate your weight automatically. Just eat, exercise, get proper sleep and your body will do the rest. You don't have to count calories or weigh portions of food. You don't need to worry about carbs, protein or fat. A whole food diet will provide everything you need automatically.

Optimum diet percentages

Important note: The percentage recommendations in this section are presented for informational completeness. They are also of value if you are using nutritional software to plan and evaluate your diet. Nutritional software is covered in chapter eleven.

The percentages can also serve as a rough guide, you can think of them when planning your meals if that will help maintain a balanced diet. If you don't like thinking about percentages, an alternative way to insure a balanced diet is to follow the sections "Balanced breakfast" at the end of chapter eight and "Balanced lunch & dinner" at the end of chapter nine.

A whole food diet worked well throughout human history, long before we had any idea of what a percentage breakdown was, so it is not mandatory to think about percentages. It is very difficult to create a nutritionally deficient whole food diet as long as you are eating a variety of foods. Portion control and calorie counting are not needed with a whole food diet, so you can put your scale away!

Where did the percentages come from? - The percentages below are a statistical average of the healthiest diets from around the world, both modern and historical. Keep in mind that the percentages are by calories and not weight. Calories are a measurement of the amount of energy that is in food. Remember that some foods have high energy levels like nuts so it does not take a lot of nuts to make up 10-35% or your total diet. On the other hand vegetables have a low energy level (but a very high level of nutrients), so to get 30-50% of your calories from vegetables you will be eating a much larger physical volume of vegetables.

- 30-50% Vegetables
- 15-35% Fruits & Berries
- 15-35% Legumes
- 15-35% Seeds & Nuts
- 5-20% Grains & Starches
- 0-10% Meat, fish and eggs (lean organic)
- 0% Processed food
- 0% Dairy

Percentages explained

Vegetables - 30-50% of your calories

Vegetables provide many of the vitamins, minerals and phytochemicals in your diet, but are low in calories. Vegetables are divided between cooked and raw. It is important to have some raw vegetables, because they are high in beneficial bacteria and other nutrients. A good balance is to eat at least 1/4 of your vegetables raw and the rest can be cooked. This is also the most comfortable way to eat for most people. While most people like some raw vegetables, they don't enjoy chomping raw veggies all day. While some nutrients in vegetables decrease with cooking, some nutrients actually increase during cooking. Cooked does not mean overcooked. Cooking lightly will retain most of the nutrients. We will go into detail about how to cook vegetables for optimum nutritional value in chapter seven.

Fruits & berries - 15-35% of your calories

Fruits & berries are high in nutrients and contain many beneficial antioxidants. The nutrients in fruits & berries complement the types of nutrients in vegetables, so both are important and you should have a balance in your diet. It is OK to have more fruit when it is in season and less at other times. If you are low on fruit just eat more vegetables to make up the difference.

Legumes - 15-35% of your calories

Legumes include beans, lentils, peas, soy and peanuts (which are technically not nuts, they are legumes). Legumes are high in protein and are an abundant source of good slow burning carbohydrates for energy. Legumes are high in fiber and complement grains as a source of complex carbohydrates.

Seeds & nuts - 15-35% of your calories

Seeds and nuts are high in some nutrients that are lacking in the other categories and are an important part of a balanced diet. Some seeds and nuts such as flaxseed and walnuts are a good source of omega 3 fatty acids.

Grains & starches - 5-20% of your calories

Grains include whole grains like oats, millet, rice, quinoa, barley and wheat berries. Starches include potatoes, yams, sweet potatoes, cassava (yuca root) and modern corn (maize). Grains and starches have lower nutrient value than legumes, but are still important to have in your diet. Grains and legumes are used together in many cuisines, in dishes such as beans and rice, tofu and rice, beans and corn, etc.

Meat, fish and eggs (organic only) - 0% to 10% of your calories

Meat, fish and eggs are optional. Some people reject all meat, fish and eggs, while others choose to retain a limited amount of lean, organically farmed meat, fish and eggs. This is a controversial subject and most people are quite polarized in their opinions. I have spent several years looking at the research to determine if I wanted to remove all meat, fish and eggs from my diet. First, I will tell you what the research says and then I will tell you my personal take at the end of the section. You can then make up your mind about whether to reject or include some meat, fish and eggs in your diet.

There are no nutrients in meat, fish and eggs that are not better obtained from plant based whole foods. Some people argue that meat is the best source of protein, but this is not the case. This will be covered in the section "Macronutrients" later in this chapter. Other people argue that meat is a vital source of vitamin D and vitamin B12. Actually, In the case of vitamin D, meat, fish and eggs contain only small amounts. Your body generates vitamin D through exposure to sunlight. In the case of vitamin B12 it comes from dirt. Meat, fish and eggs only contain B12 because the animals ate dirt with their food, animals do not generate their own B12. We will talk in detail about vitamins D and B12 in the section "Special considerations" later in this chapter.

As we talked about earlier in the chapter, historically the vast majority of humans had a whole food diet with low to moderate meat consumption. The meat was very lean and free from contaminants. Because the meat, fish and eggs that are available today have higher levels of contaminants (even organically farmed) it is advisable to reduce our consumption of meat, fish or eggs from historical levels, or eliminate meat completely.

The large scale research data clearly supports reducing meat, fish and eggs to less than 10% of your diet or eliminating meat, fish and eggs entirely. There are studies showing that some amount of animal based products may be beneficial, but these studies are questionable because the food industry is actively funding the research. It is telling that the large scale studies show that reducing or eliminating meat, fish and eggs is better for health, while the smaller studies that are funded by the food industry always show the opposite.

The recommendation of 0-10% is based on lean, organically farmed meat, fish and eggs. If you are consuming factory farmed meat, fish and eggs, you should keep the total percentage to under 5%, but it is best to abstain completely from factory farmed meat, fish and eggs. Keep in mind that the recommended percentage is by calories and not weight. Since meat, fish and eggs are high in calories, the amount it takes to get to 5% or 10% or your total calories is relatively small.

My personal preference is to eat only lean, organically farmed meat, fish and eggs and to limit them to less than 2% of my diet. Looking back on the last 5 years my consumption has been under 2% and most of this is from sardines. Some people with cancer choose to eliminate all animal products from their diet, because there is research that shows that animal products feed cancer at any level of consumption. I tend to agree with this. If I had cancer, or any serious medical condition for that matter, I would immediately eliminate all animal products from my diet.

Since meat, fish and eggs bring no nutritional benefit to a whole food diet the consideration of whether to include them in your diet should be a simple one between the health concerns and any culinary value that meat, fish and eggs may hold for you.

Dairy - 0% of your calories

I am not happy about the recommendation that follows, because I like the taste of cheese and other dairy products. I still use a small amount of half & half in my coffee sometimes, because I have tried every other type of coffee creamer available and nothing comes close to half & half. Eventually I will stop using it as well. Even though I really like cheese and a few other dairy products, I have made the choice that my health must come first.

My recommendation is to eliminate dairy from your diet. There are no nutrients in dairy that are not better obtained from plant based whole foods. The research supporting the elimination of dairy products is overwhelming. There was no dairy in our historical diet, before animals were domesticated. Our bodies are not designed for dairy. There are no animals except humans that consume the milk from another species. Even humans stop consuming their mothers milk at an early age. Milk is designed to cause rapid cell growth and weight gain in babies. In adults milk feeds the growth of cancer cells, exactly what we don't want. Dairy also promotes diseases such as heart disease and osteoporosis. The effects of dairy on our health is covered in detail in chapter two.

Processed foods - 0% of your calories

My recommendation is to eliminate all processed foods from your diet. There are no nutrients in processed foods that are not better obtained from whole foods. The research supporting the elimination of processed food is overwhelming. Processed food promotes disease and obesity. There was no processed food in our historical diet, our bodies were not designed for processed food. Processed food is addictive. It is hard to eat just a little processed food, so it is best to eliminate processed food all together. The effects of processed foods on our health is covered in detail in chapter two.

Macronutrients (Carbs, Protein, Fat, Fiber, Water)

Macro means large, so macronutrients are nutrients that you eat in large amounts. They are what powers your body. Macronutrients also have other roles, such as helping to build muscle cells. The five types of macronutrients are carbohydrates, protein, fat, fiber and water.

With a balanced whole food diet you will get the correct amount of macronutrients automatically. You don't need to keep track of them or to do anything special. There are many misconceptions about protein, fat and carbohydrates. Most of these misconceptions are promoted by the food and supplement industries to sell products. I will deconstruct some of them later in this chapter.

Carbohydrates

Carbohydrates provide energy and perform other chemical signaling functions that are just starting to be understood. There are two types of carbohydrates, refined carbohydrates (also known as simple carbohydrates) and complex carbohydrates. All of the bad things that you may have read about carbohydrates are referring to the refined type, such as sugar and high fructose corn syrup. Refined carbohydrates are a primary ingredient in most processed foods. There are many tricky names that the food industry uses for refined carbohydrates, some "sugar free" processed foods actually contain refined carbohydrates! In a whole food diet there are no refined carbohydrates, so by eliminating processed food from your diet you have also eliminated any concerns about refined carbohydrates.

Complex carbohydrates are a vital source of short term energy for your body and are healthy. This is the type of carbohydrate you get in a whole food diet. The bottom line is that with a whole food diet you can stop worrying about carbs, no need to count calories. You will automatically get the right type and the right amount that your body needs.

Protein

Protein is used by your body for antibodies, collagen, elastin, lean muscle tissue and many other functions. The misconception that vegetables can't provide the complete protein your body needs is widespread. All protein is broken down by your digestive system into the basic building blocks (amino acids) before it is absorbed by your body. These building blocks are then assembled by your body into complete proteins as they are needed. A balanced whole food diet provides all of the protein you need, meat is not necessary. In fact protein from plant based whole foods is superior to protein from meat, fish, eggs or dairy, because plant based whole foods have lower levels of unwanted chemicals, pesticides, antibiotics, hormones and other contaminants.

I am always surprised by how many people think that meat is protein. When they see me with a big plate of vegetables they will ask "Where is your protein?" (meaning where is my meat). I explain that vegetables have plenty of protein and that although meat has protein too, meat is not the same thing as protein!

To put the plant protein issue to rest once and for all, I asked several nutritionists using advanced software to intentionally design a whole food diet that is protein deficient. They couldn't do it. No reasonable whole food diet they could construct was even close to being protein deficient. In chapter eleven several sources of nutritional analysis software are listed. This software includes a full food composition database. You can run this test yourself if you have any lingering concerns. The bottom line is that with a whole food diet you can stop worrying about protein, you will get the amount of protein that your body needs.

Eating extra protein has no benefit, because your body cannot store protein. Extra protein is converted by your body into ATP (adenosine triphosphate, a form of chemical energy) during the TCA cycle (tricarboxylic acid cycle, one of the cycles of your metabolism). ATP is used to power your body or is converted to fat and stored, if your body is not in need of immediate energy. Eating extra protein can be unhealthy. If you eat extra protein you are altering the ratio between fat, carbs and protein that your body was designed for. Anytime you deviate from the natural ratio, it causes problems and inefficiencies, just like if you put the wrong type of fuel into your car.

Carbohydrates are the preferred source of energy to power your body, followed by fat. Protein is the least preferred source, because your body has to expend extra energy and fluids to process the protein into energy. The energy spent on processing protein is energy that is lost! Even if you are an Olympic athlete or an Olympic powerlifter, a whole food diet will provide all of the protein you need. We will cover protein for athletes and go into more detail about misconceptions concerning protein in chapter ten.

Fat

Fat is a source of long term energy and is used for storing energy in your body. Fatty acids also have many other roles in the body, such as serving as the building blocks for cell membranes, immune regulators, nerve sheaths and hormones.

There are several different types of fats such as monounsaturated fat, polyunsaturated fat, saturated fat, trans fat and unsaturated fat. Trans fat is bad for health and causes heart disease. Saturated fat has also been found to promote heart disease. Animal fat is high in saturated fat.

Keeping track of all these types of fats is complicated. Fortunately with a whole food diet you don't need to worry about fat, you will automatically get the right amount of fat and the right kinds of fat that your body needs. The only exception is that you need to have sufficient quantities of omega 3 and this can come from flaxseed, walnuts or fish. This is covered in the section "Special considerations" later in this chapter. One more consideration about fat is that you do need to be sensible with nuts and nut butter. If you unbalance your diet and eat huge amounts of nuts (or peanut butter) you could gain weight.

Fiber

Dietary fiber (often called roughage) aids the digestive process and has several other roles such as the absorption of chemicals and water. The American diet is deficient in fiber and causes chronic constipation and promotes colon cancer. Dietary fiber is plentiful in whole foods. With a whole food diet you will automatically get the right amount of dietary fiber that your body needs. You can put the fiber supplements and laxatives in the trash!

Water

Water is used as a transport fluid for most bodily functions and is a solvent for the chemical reactions that sustain life. Water also plays many other roles as an essential nutrient. In the section "Special considerations" later in this chapter we will go over how much water you need on a daily basis.

You need the right amount of water. Too little water and you dehydrate, too much and your body must labor to remove it. In cooler climates without vigorous exercise, most medium sized people need 1.25 liters of water per day (5 US cups). Small people need 1 liter (4 cups), large people need 1.75 liters (7 cups). More water is needed with vigorous exercise or in hot climates. More water is needed for pregnant women and women that are breastfeeding. Drinking large amounts of water for no reason, puts extra stress on your kidneys and has no medical benefit. Fad water drinking recommendations (such as 8 to 12 cups a day) have no medical basis. That being said, you should let your body guide you, if you are thirsty and feel dehydrated, then drink.

The amount of water you drink depends on the amount of water you are getting in your food. Some types of food like watermelon are mostly water. If your urine is dark colored and you urinate infrequently you should drink more water. If your urine is clear and your are urinating very frequently you may be drinking too much water. For more information about hydration, including during extended exercise, or for very hot weather conditions, see the section on water in chapter ten.

Micronutrients (Vitamins & Minerals)

Micro means small, so micronutrients are nutrients that you eat in small quantities. Even though you only eat small quantities, they are very important. Micronutrients include vitamins, minerals and phytochemicals.

The important thing to know, is that a whole food diet provides all of the micronutrients that you need with only two possible exceptions, D3 and B12. That is the beauty of a balanced whole food diet, it provides the high quality vitamins, minerals, flavonoids, antioxidants and phytochemicals that you need. Because of this and for the sake of keeping it simple, we will not go over a long list of vitamins. If you have an interest in macronutrients, Wikipedia has a tremendous amount of information and is more up to date the most books on the subject.

Throw your vitamins in the trash, including multivitamins. Taking unneeded vitamins can damage your health and confuse the systems in your body. Taking large quantities of nutrients that have been chemically removed from their source foods deviates from the natural balance of nutrients that your body is expecting. If you are eating a balanced whole food diet, adding more vitamins and minerals is not better, and will only hurt you. This may be counter-intuitive and hard for people to understand, because in the modern consumer mindset more is always better. In the case of vitamins more is not better, more is unhealthy.

If you are sick and you think that vitamin C will help, eat oranges or papaya! This is the form of vitamin C that your body was made to utilize, not vitamins from a pill that are processed and refined to high densities in a factory. If you are concerned with nutrients, learn which foods have high amounts of the nutrient you want, and eat more of these foods.

Special considerations

When eating a balanced diet of whole foods based on modern varieties of vegetables and fruit that are currently available in our food supply system, there are only four special concerns that should be addressed. These are sodium, vitamin D, vitamin B12 and omega 3 fatty acid.

Sodium and iodine

You need the right amount of sodium. Too much sodium causes health problems such as high blood pressure. Too little sodium also causes health problems such as dizziness or feeling weak. A sodium deficiency can cause you to have a heat stroke. If you are not sweating much, the right amount of sodium is 1500 mg to 1800 per day during winter and 1800 mg - 2000 mg per day during summer. If you are doing vigorous exercise, are in a hot climate or are sweating a lot you should increase your sodium intake. The sodium that is naturally in the foods you eat should be included along with the sodium that is added to your food to arrive at your total sodium intake. For information about how to increase your sodium intake for athletes and other people doing extended exercise, or for very hot weather conditions, see the section on salt in chapter ten.

Table salt is comprised of about 40% sodium based on weight. This means that one teaspoon of table salt has about 2300 mg of sodium. Based on the foods in your diet, you should calculate the amount of sodium you are getting from food and drinks and subtract that from your target sodium intake to find the amount of sodium to add to your food. For example: lets say your target is 1800 mg and you are eating all fresh foods with no canned food. In this case you may be getting about 650 mg of sodium from your food, so you should add ½ teaspoon of iodized table salt to arrive at about 1800 mg of sodium total. On days when you have heavy athletic activity, add some additional sodium to your drinking water as described in chapter 10. Your day to day sodium intake does not have to be exact, anything between 1500 to 2200 is fine, older people generally need a little more sodium than younger people.

Most table salt is fortified with iodine, this is known as iodized salt. Some brands of sea salt are also fortified with iodine. You should always use iodized salt unless you are sure that you are eating foods that provide enough iodine to meet your daily requirements or are taking iodine separately. Most foods do not have sufficient quantities to meet the daily requirements. Iodine is a mineral that comes from the soil, many farms have soil that is deficient in iodine, so the foods that are grown are also deficient. An iodine deficient diet causes a condition known as goiter which usually results in an enlarged thyroid gland. The recommended daily requirement for iodine is 150 micrograms (0.15 mg) per day.

Vitamin D3

Vitamin D3 is created by your body through the exposure of your skin to the sun, but many people in modern society stay indoors and do not get sufficient exposure to the sun. Most people take 400 I.U. to 2000 I.U. of vitamin D3 per day depending on age and sun exposure. If you get a lot of exposure to the sun, you do not need to take as much vitamin D3. If you are older you need slightly more vitamin D3. Vitamin D3 comes in the form of a vitamin pill. Don't take large quantities of vitamin D, you need the right amount, not large amounts. Vitamin D can be toxic in large quantities.

Vitamin B12

Vitamin B12 comes from bacteria in dirt, but in modern societies we wash our foods quite well and may not consume enough dirt to get the proper amount of B12. With the widespread use of chemical fertilizers and pesticides, not washing away the dirt would be a bad idea unless you are eating organic food. Some meat has vitamin B12, because the animals ate dirt while eating grass or other food. Not all meat has significant quantities of vitamin B12. Some meat from factory farmed animals is deficient in B12, because the animals are fed processed animal food that does not have dirt in it. Most people should take vitamin B12 in the form of a vitamin pill or in the form of nutritional yeast that is available through some grocery stores. Red Star is a popular brand of nutritional yeast. Red Star makes a Vegetarian Support Formula that has consistent amounts of vitamin B12. 1-1/2 tablespoons a day is the amount that most people take. Vitamin B12 is also present in fortified soy milk.

Recommended intake for vitamin B12 ranges from 1.5 MCG in the UK to 7 MCG per day according to some recent studies in the US. The reason why most people take a 500 MCG or 1000 MCG vitamin B12 pill is that the digestive absorption rate is only around 1%. This means that if you take 500 MCG of vitamin B12 only 5 MCG should be absorbed, but not so fast! To further complicate the issue, there is a limit to how much vitamin B12 can be absorbed orally at one time. This is about 1.5 MCG. Because of this it makes sense to split your intake between two lower doses taken at different times of the day. Another factor is that older people have a reduced ability to absorb vitamin B12. If you are concerned about your vitamin B12 level it is relatively inexpensive to have it tested. Fortunately your body stores enough B12 for several years, so the concerns are long term, a few days or weeks of missed B12 has no effect on healthy people. The Wikipedia entry for vitamin B12 has a lot of good information if you want to do further reading.

Personally, I take vitamin B12 from two sources and at different times during the day. This usually consists of nutritional yeast on my oatmeal for breakfast and a 500 MCG pill after dinner. Sometimes I also use some nutritional yeast or vitamin B12 fortified soy milk at lunch in my smoothie.

Omega 3

Omega 3 fatty acids are important building blocks for heart muscle cells and brain cells. Making sure you get enough omega 3's is easy, because there are several foods that are high in omega 3 such as flaxseed, walnuts, chia, hemp, sesame and fish. Two tablespoons (14g) of ground flaxseed will provide enough omega 3 to meet your daily requirement. You can add this to your oatmeal or to any other dish. One ounce (28g) of walnuts will also give you enough omega 3. If you want to get technical and are tracking your diet with nutritional software, the ratio of omega 6 to omega 3 preferably should be less than 8 to 1, optimally about 4 to 1.

Frequently Asked Questions

Question: This is all overwhelming. Eat this, don't eat that, this is toxic, that's not. How can a person live their life worrying about all this? This is enough to drive a person crazy!

Answer: The best plan is to prioritize. Identify the top dietary concerns and address those first. Deal with as many as you can comfortably, without becoming a nut case. After you master the most important things, then you can identify less important items to attack over time, when you are ready.

Start simple and do it in steps:

1. Learn to shop for whole foods and start cooking with whole foods.
2. Eat a balanced assortment of whole foods.
3. Drop processed food and factory farmed animal products from your diet.
4. Make sure you are getting your B12, D3 and Omega 3.
5. Get proper sleep and exercise.
6. Over time learn to prepare better dishes, if you are not happy with what you are able to prepare.
7. Over time start taking toxins into account. Look at sites like www.EWG.org to see which foods to avoid. This is explained in chapter five.
8. Identify other areas you want to improve and make your own priority list.

Don't do it all at once, go at a comfortable pace. Just rejecting the American diet and switching to a whole food diet makes a huge improvement. The rest are additional improvements that will add up over time, but the most significant thing is to make the jump to a whole food diet.

Question: Does it matter what time of day you eat? Also, I like to eat late at night, I have heard this is not good.

Answer: Eating a good diet is far more important than when you eat. In general you should eat 3 times a day or more so your body is able to have a flow of energy from the food you are eating. If you eat 4 or 5 times a day, some of the times you eat can be a snack, like some fruit. It is better to spread your food out over 3 meals then to have 1 big meal. Eating a large meal late at night, right before you go to sleep is not a good idea because it can give you painful gas or other digestive issues. Motion and activity are a needed part of your digestion process and your system does not perform well if you are laying down immediately after eating a large meal.

Question: What do you think about calorie restricted diets?

Answer: Cutting unneeded calories from your diet will increase your life expectancy and slow aging. During the great depression in the late 1920's in the United States the life expectancy increased due to calorie restriction. Unneeded calories feed diseases such as cancer and Alzheimer's. Calorie restriction should not be confused with starvation however, and a body mass index of about 20 or more should be maintained. There is research being done presently in this area. This is something that I intend to look into, and possibly write about.

Question: What about Selenium?

Answer: Selenium is a chemical element that is a necessary part of our diet. A balanced whole food diet will normally provide all of the selenium you need. There is ongoing research trying to define the role of selenium in fighting diseases such as cancer and HIV. If you have concerns about getting enough selenium you can always eat a Brazil nut every day. One single Brazil nut has more than the recommended daily allowance of selenium!

Question: What about Choline?

Answer: Choline is a nutrient that is grouped with the B-complex vitamins. It is a necessary part of your diet. A balanced whole food diet will normally provide all of the Choline you need. Some endurance athletes take Choline supplements, but this is unnecessary if sufficient quantities of cruciferous (green leafy) vegetables are eaten.

Question: What about DHA, Antioxidants, Phytochemicals, Coenzyme Q10, Vitamin E, L-Carnitine, Protein, etc, etc, etc.

Answer: A balanced whole food diet provides all of these things. The beauty of a balanced whole food diet is that you don't need to worry about getting enough nutrients. If you just want to worry (and some people do), do your research and eat the natural foods that are high in the nutrients you are concerned with. This is a much better approach than buying a supplement of unknown origin or quality from a company that is part of an industry with little or no regulation. Many vitamin and supplement sellers look very credible, but looks mean little or nothing. Making supplements is a complicated process involving chemicals from many suppliers. Even well meaning supplement manufacturers do not have control over all of the chemicals that are used in their products. The fact that supplements now cause over 20 percent of all liver damage in the United States proves this point. Supplement sellers are not your friends, they are in business to make a profit. If they were your friends they would advise you to eat whole foods and leave the supplements alone!

5 - A Look at Whole Foods

In this chapter we will get acquainted with the foods that make up a whole food diet. As we go through the foods we will point out some of the nutrients and disease fighting capabilities. Keep in mind that all whole foods are nutrient rich and contribute to your health. At the end of the chapter we will cover GMO, organics, cage free & free range, wild food and how to reduce food toxins.

Most varieties of fruits and vegetables available in stores were domesticated (bred) from wild varieties thousands of years ago. If you are curious about the effects of breeding and want to compare the original and domesticated varieties, a good book on the subject is "Eating on the Wild Side" by Jo Robinson.

Vegetables

Alliums - Alliums are commonly called onions and include several types. Onions have alliinase enzymes that fights cancer cell growth. Western Yellow onions are the most nutritious type of onion, followed by Red onions. Common types of alliums include: Onion, Garlic, Leek, Chive, Shallot, Scallion and Green onion.

Herbs & Spices - Herbs and spices are not just for seasoning, most herbs and spices have disease fighting nutrients. Common types of herbs and spices include: Mint, Dill, Turmeric, Fennel, Rosemary, Basil, Tea Leaf, Thyme, Lavender, Coriander, Paprika and Ginger.

Leaf Vegetables - Leaf vegetables are the largest source of phytochemicals, antioxidants and cancer fighting nutrients in a whole food diet. For maximum nutritional benefit a major part of your vegetables (300 calories or more) should be in the form of dark green leafy vegetables such as Collard greens or Kale. It is best to combine two or more different types. You don't have to eat large amounts of uncooked leaf vegetables (salad) unless you like to, because there are many ways to prepare and cook leaf vegetables. Common types of leaf vegetables include: Collard greens, Kale, Mustard greens, Turnip greens, Watercress, Spinach, Swiss chard, Bok choy, Arugula, Cilantro, Parsley, Cabbage, Brussels sprouts, Romaine Lettuce, Napa Cabbage, Broccoli, Cauliflower and Iceberg lettuce.

Mushrooms - Mushrooms have many immune system building nutrients that are just now being discovered. The nutrients in mushrooms help prevent abnormal cell growth. Mushrooms contain some types of phytochemicals that are not found in other vegetables. Mushrooms can be mixed with other foods or used separately as a side dish. Common types of mushrooms include: Shiitake, Portobello, Cremini, White, Brown and Oyster.

Peppers - Peppers are great cooked or raw. Red bell peppers are far more nutritious than green ones and contain the antioxidant lycopene and high amounts of vitamin C. Common types of peppers include: Red bell pepper, Green bell pepper and Chili pepper.

Root Vegetables - If you buy root vegetables with their green stalks and tops attached, they will be fresh, if you buy them without the tops they may be more than two months old. Freezing destroys some of the nutrients in root vegetables. In some places you can find purple carrots, they are more nutritious than orange carrots. Avoid baby carrots, they are actually not babies, they are full grown carrots that are cut to size, the outer part that is thrown away is the most nutritious part. Cooking will cause most root vegetables to gain nutritional value, because cooking breaks down the cell structure and makes the nutrients more bio available. Common types of root vegetables include: Carrot, Beet, Turnip, Rutabaga, Radish and Parsnip.

Sea Vegetables - Sea vegetables can be mixed with other foods to add flavor and texture, or use them as a side dish. Sea vegetables have many nutrients including iodine, thiamine, calcium, sea salt and niacin. Wakame is one of the few green vegetables with high levels of omega 3 fatty acid. In the US the most common source of sea vegetables is through Asian food stores, large packages of dried wakame and kombu are available inexpensively. Sea vegetables make an excellent flavoring for soups and seafood dishes such as clam chowder. Common types of sea vegetables include: Wakame, Kombu and Nori.

Squashes - Squashes have a long shelf life and are great when you want a change of pace. They can be used in place of yams or potatoes. Common types of squashes include: Pumpkin, Cucumber, Zucchini, Yellow Squash, Eggplant and Acorn squash.

Tomato - Lycopene is a serious cancer fighting nutrient. Tomatoes are a good source of lycopene, but nothing is better than tomato sauce and tomato paste which have 3 to 10 times as much lycopene as any other natural source.

Wild Plants & Weeds - Many types of wild plants and weeds are higher in nutritional value than domesticated vegetables. They are also free and add variety to your diet. Purslane is a nutritional powerhouse and grows almost everywhere in the world. Palmer Amaranth is a wild leafy green plant that was cultivated and eaten by native American Indians. It is now considered a weed in the United States and is resistant to the GMO pesticide Roundup. Alarmists think that Palmer Amaranth could threaten the modern food supply, but it is actually far more nutritious than the GMO crops. A better idea would be to grow palmer amaranth like the Indians did. Then the farmers wouldn't need to buy Roundup! Common types of wild plants and weeds include: Purslane, Dandelion, Amaranth, Chickweed, Tart greens, Wintercress and Garlic mustard.

Fruits & Berries

Berries - All berries are high in nutrients, blueberries and other dark skinned berries are highest in disease fighting nutrients. Berries are not available all year round, but frozen berries are always available and berries do not lose much nutritional value when frozen. If you thaw frozen berries in the microwave, they retain twice as much of the nutrient value compared to slowly thawing them. Frozen berries are less expensive than fresh berries. Common types of berries include: Blackberry, Blueberry, Boysenberry, Cranberry, Huckleberry, Raspberry, Mulberry and Strawberry.

Citrus Fruit - Suppliers often use ethylene gas to change the color of fruit from green to orange, red or yellow to hide the fact that they are really not ripe. This is why some fruit that looks ripe really is not ripe and tastes bitter. Before buying a lot of fruit, buy a piece and try it first, this is the best way to tell if the fruit was force ripened. Another option is to buy organic. Organic fruit is not supposed to be force ripened. Common types of citrus fruit include: Orange, Grapefruit, Lemon and lime.

Melons - Melons are great to eat in the summer, but have less nutritional value than other fruits. As a rule the varieties with darker inside flesh have more nutritional value. Common types of melons include: Watermelon, Cantaloupe, Casaba, Winter melon and Honeydew.

Tree Fruit - Try to buy organic tree fruit, otherwise they are heavily sprayed with pesticides and may be forced ripened. Organic tree fruit is ugly and has more blemishes from insects and fungus, but that is OK, it is better than pristine looking fruit that is saturated with pesticides. Also organic fruit is generally not waxed, the wax will trap the pesticides and eating wax is not healthy. Most of the nutrients are in the skins of tree fruits such as apples, pears and plums, so eat the skins if they are organic. Common types of tree fruit include: Apple, Pear, Apricot, Cherry, Peach, Plum and Rose Hip.

Tropical Fruit - Of the tropical fruits mangos, guavas, papayas and avocado are the most nutritious and have the least sugar content, if they are in season they should be your first choice. Common types of tropical fruit include: Avocado, Pineapple, Banana, Plantain, Mango, Guava, Coconut, Passion fruit, Papayas, Breadfruit and Jackfruit.

Vine Fruit - Black and red grapes are more nutritious than thompson grapes or white grapes. Common types of vine fruit include: Grape, Kiwi, Raisin and Currant.

Legumes

Legumes - Legumes should supply a lot of your carbohydrates and protein. Nutritionally legumes complement leafy green vegetables, together they provide a large part of your total nutritional requirements. The type of carbs that are in legumes take a long time to digest, so they will give you energy for many hours and keep you from getting hungry. When you do start to run out of energy, it will happen very slowly. Desi chickpeas are dark colored and smaller in size than the more common tan chickpeas, and they are three times more nutritious. Common types of legumes include: Lentil, Lima bean, Chickpea, Desi chickpea, Pinto bean, Black bean, Green pea, Soybean, Tofu, Edamame, Kidney bean, Black eyed pea, Fava bean, Green bean, Snap pea, Snow pea and Mung bean.

Seeds & Nuts

Nuts - Some nuts have high nutritional value, such as walnuts and hazelnuts. Walnuts are high in omega 3 fatty acids. Eating a lot of nuts can cause you to gain weight, so it is best to include nuts in your meals and not just eat nuts separately as a snack food unless you are hiking and need the energy. Technically peanuts are a legume, but they are nutritionally closer to nuts, so they are commonly categorized as a nut. Some stores have grinders in the bulk food department for making peanut butter and almond butter so that you can grind it yourself. The resulting nut butter is fresh and free from unwanted ingredients. The processed nut butters sold in most stores (in jars) have unwanted ingredients such as palm oil and may be many months old. Common types of nuts include: Walnut, Hazelnut, Peanut, Almond, Brazil nut, Pecan and Cashew.

Seeds - Seeds were designed to have concentrated nutrients to facilitate the reproduction of plants, they also have several types of beneficial fats not found elsewhere in high concentration. Chia and flax seed are high in omega 3 fatty acids. Some seeds such as flax seeds must be ground, because your digestive system can not break down the tough outer hull (shell). If you eat the whole seed, it will pass right through you undigested, giving you no nutritional benefit. Always buy ground flax seed unless you are going to grind your own. Common types of seeds include: Flaxseed, Sesame, Hemp seed, Chia and Sunflower seeds.

Grains & Starches

Grains - Oats are a winner with many disease fighting qualities. They also are a good source of complex carbs to give you long term energy. For this reason they are a favorite breakfast food (oatmeal) that can power you through the day. Oats have the highest protein content of all grains at 12% to 24% depending on the type. Other types of grains are also good as an alternative to oatmeal for breakfast.

Rice like most grains has an outer covering (husk), an inner covering (bran), a starchy part (endosperm) and a center kernel (germ). Brown rice is unmilled rice that has the husk removed, but the bran and germ are still intact. White rice goes through a milling process to remove the bran and germ leaving only the starchy endosperm. This makes white rice far less nutritious than brown rice. Parboiled rice is partially boiled while in the husk. This causes most of the nutrients from the bran and germ to migrate to the endosperm, so parboiled rice retains 80% of the nutrients of brown rice. Brown rice and parboiled rice are nutritionally superior to white rice. White rice should be considered a processed food and avoided. All rice contains trace amounts of arsenic. Normally this does not pose a problem, but you should limit rice consumption to less than one cup per day of cooked rice.

Buckwheat is a completely different species from regular wheat, it only has wheat in the name. Kasha is buckwheat that has been toasted. Buckwheat cooks quickly and can be used for soups, salads, granola, hot cereals, etc.

What about gluten? Gluten is not a concern with a whole food diet, unless you actually have celiac disease and only a very small percentage of people have it. Most people that think they have celiac disease actually have other digestive issues caused by processed foods that have nothing to do with gluten. Even people who have a problem with processed gluten may not have a problem with the gluten in natural unprocessed whole grains. Processing concentrates the gluten and turns it into something unnatural. If there is a concern, wheat, barley and rye can simply be avoided. There are plenty of other grains to choose from.

Common types of grains include: Brown rice, Parboiled rice, Oatmeal, Wheat berries, Barley, Corn, Millet, Rye, Quinoa, Sorghum, Buckwheat and bulgur wheat.

Tubers - Potatoes should be bought organically if possible. Most potatoes are frequently sprayed with pesticides and fungicides and are also sprayed with sprout inhibiting chemicals. The russet burbank type of potato has the more nutrients than other common types of potatoes. The yams and sweet potatoes sold in grocery stores, are actually slightly different versions of the same species. They have less carbs and more nutrients than modern types of potatoes. Cassava is a common staple food in much of the world and is a good alternative to other tubers because of the distinctive flavor and texture. Common types of tubers include: Yam, Potato, Sweet potato, Yuca root (Cassava) and Taro.

Soy based foods

Soy sauce - Make sure to only use naturally brewed soy sauce. Chemically derived soy sauce is made using toxic chemicals that are not totally removed during processing. All soy sauce has acrylamide, a known carcinogen. I love soy sauce, but because of the acrylamide issue, I limit my use to a couple times a week in moderation.

Tempeh - Tempeh is made from fermented whole soybeans and can take the form of blocks, cake or patties. Some types of tempeh are made from a mix of soy and other types of beans and grains. Since tempeh is made with whole beans, it has a higher amount of nutrients than tofu. Tempeh has a nutty mushroom like flavor and can be eaten as-is or cooked.

Tofu - Tofu (also called bean curd), is made of coagulated soy milk that is pressed into blocks. Tofu does not occur naturally and is a lightly processed food, but it does not have a substantially increased energy density and is considered to be acceptable by most people with a whole food diet. Tofu comes in a few consistencies, very soft, soft, medium, firm and extra firm. Tofu can be cut into cubes and served without cooking, it is often eaten with soy sauce or other flavorings. Tofu may also be fried or baked. Tofu does not have a strong flavor and when cooked, tofu absorbs flavorings well, so it can taste many different ways depending on how you season it. Organic tofu is not much more expensive than regular tofu, sometimes the cost is the same.

Animal Based Foods

Since better quality nutrients are found in plant based whole foods, eating animal based foods is optional. If you do eat animal based foods, it is best to eat a variety and not just one type. By eating a variety of animal products from different sources you will reduce the degree of exposure to any one type of toxin (such as antibiotics, hormones, mercury or PCB's).

Eggs - Try to limit consumption of eggs to a few a week, or just eliminate them. There is no nutritional necessity to eat eggs and negative health impacts are a concern. Standards like cage free and free range are marketing terms with little meaning. Most commercially farmed chickens are de-beaked and live in enclosures so small, that they can't flap their wings. Standards like Certified Humane and Certified Organic are somewhat more stringent, but still lacking.

Fish - Most farmed fish, especially salmon, is high in toxins such as dioxin and PCB's, in fact many times higher than factory farmed beef. Mercury can be a problem in fish from any source. Take the time and do your research. There are several web sites that can make this easier, they are listed in chapter twelve. Recent DNA testing of fish sold in restaurants and stores has found that many types of fish are fraudulently sold as a different species. Some species such as tuna and red snapper are mislabeled 57% to 80% of the time. This presents a problem when trying to buy a specific species of fish to reduce toxins. Common types of fish include: Salmon, Tilapia, Carp, Catfish, Tuna, Sardines, Sturgeon and Halibut.

Insects - If you look at insects from a nutritional and economic perspective, they appear to be superior to other types of meat, although more testing and research in this area is needed. Insects are eaten in many countries around the world. Insect meal is also used in some processed foods, so you could be eating insects already without knowing it. In the future I plan to do more research on insects and who knows, perhaps someday I will be intentionally eating them.

Meat - Fowl is healthier than red meat (beef). Take the time to ask questions and research where your meat is coming from. If you buy from local farms, sometimes it is possible to go visit the farm yourself. The book "The End of Dieting" by Joel Fuhrman M.D. has a lot of scientifically backed information about the health concerns for meat and animal products. Avoid animal organs such as liver and kidneys, because they have much higher levels of toxins including heavy metals. These organs perform a filtering function that causes them to collect toxins. Common types of meat include: Chicken, Turkey, Beef, Pork, Bison, Venison, Emu and Ostrich.

Seafood - Toxins are a concern with seafood. There are several sites on the internet that list toxin levels in seafood and fish, it's a good idea to look at one of these sites before buying seafood. Common types of seafood include: Clams, Oysters, Mussels, Scallops, Octopus, Squid, Snails, Abalone, Cuttlefish, Crab, Shrimp, Prawns and Crayfish.

Alternatives to meat

For many years the meat industry has promoted meat as the centerpiece most meals. It will take time to change from this way of thinking. Make vegetables the centerpiece and use meat as a side item or eliminate it from your diet. Some people use Tofu, Tempeh, Hummus, Peanut butter, Almond butter or Texturized vegetable protein as a substitute for meat. The quicker you stop thinking of meat as the centerpiece the better, at that point you will no longer need to find alternatives to meat.

Sweeteners

Some people put sugar on foods such as rice, potatoes, oatmeal, green vegetables, ice tea, etc. This is a tough habit to break. Unfortunately, there are people who grew up doing this from childhood, because some mothers thought this was a good way to get children to eat their vegetables! If you are having trouble with this, cut the sugar for a few months and give your taste a chance to re-calibrate. This is much better than using artificial sweeteners. If you use sweeteners you are only extending the problem.

If you do need to sweeten something, use frozen concentrated juice or some type of fruit. This is the natural solution. Do not use artificial sweeteners. Artificial sweeteners are a processed food and have many negative health impacts. Don't be fooled, every few years a new artificial sweetener is introduced that is claimed to be safe, only to be proven carcinogenic or toxic later after the public has been using it. There are no good shortcuts, bite the bullet and reprogram your taste. Once you have adjusted to a whole food diet without sweeteners, foods that are high in sugar will give you a nauseous sensation. This is what is supposed to happen if your body is not desensitized from eating foods high in sugar.

Oil

Oil is a processed food and a form of fat. This includes olive oil, extra virgin olive oil, coconut oil or whatever the latest popular oil happens to be, it is all processed and it is all a fat! Oil that is marketed as "healthy oil" with terms like "natural" or "expeller pressed" are still just oil and are still a processed food. The food industry wants you to think that some types of oil are healthy and good, like olive oil, grapeseed oil or canola oil. The biggest problem is that oil has an unnaturally high energy density with almost no nutritional value. Eating oil will alter your energy balance and cause you to gain weight. Even if it was kale oil it wouldn't change this.

Bottom line is that oil has no nutritional benefit, it is not a necessary part of a healthy diet. Whole foods have more than enough natural fats to supply all of the fat that you need in your diet. In chapter seven we will talk about cooking without oil or with small amounts of oil.

Flour

Standard commercial and general purpose flour is made by grinding grains or legumes into fine particles or powder. Most commercial flour is degerminated and heat processed at very high temperatures using steel roller mills. The germ is the most nutritious part of the grain, but is removed in general purpose flour, because natural oils in the germ go bad over time, and shorten the shelf life of the flour. All standard general purpose flours are processed foods with an increased energy density level and should be avoided.

Stone ground whole grain flour is a lightly processed food and should be used in moderation. The stone grinding wheels don't get hot, so the flour is not exposed to damaging high temperatures. Whole grain flour contains the germ and has a limited shelf life of about 6 months unless preservatives are added. If you are going to use flour, get your flour from a company that specialized in organic stone ground whole grain flours without added preservatives or other unwanted ingredients. Some companies that specialize in organic stone ground whole grain flour are listed in chapter six. Baking with stone ground whole grain flour is much different than general purpose flour, you will probably need to get new recipes or to substantially alter existing recipes.

Whole food vs health food

Most grocery stores have a health food section. Health food sections have cookies, crackers, breads and other foods that are similar to regular American processed foods, but sold under different brands that are supposedly healthier. They may be slightly healthier (or not), but are still processed foods and should be avoided. It does not make sense to replace processed foods with other slightly less processed foods. Processed foods should be eliminated and replaced by whole foods.

GMO

GMO stands for genetically modified organism. Genetically modified food is a very complicated subject that is surrounded by fear and controversy. Proponents of GMO foods claim that they are safe and present no danger. Opponents have many arguments against GMO foods. There is also an ongoing controversy about requirements to disclose GMO's on food labels.

My thoughts are that GMO foods represent a serious problem in ways that may not seem obvious. The GMO foods on the market today do not appear to present an immediate threat to human health, but there are many other factors at work. GMO's are the intellectual property of the corporations who develop them. Because GMO's are patentable, the food industry is building a large portfolio of this intellectual property. They are using this intellectual property to take control of factory farming and block new entrants into the field. This technology is still in its infancy. Having powerful technology owned and controlled by an industry that has demonstrated a long track record of putting profits over the people is a bad idea.

Organic

Organic farming is farming that promotes ecological balance and increased biodiversity. Environmentally damaging chemical fertilizers and synthetic pesticides are not used in organic farming although some pesticides may be used in special situations. Organic farming uses crop rotation and healthy organic fertilizers like manure. Cover crops are used to protect the soil and promote the growth of microbes. Organic farming requires less irrigation, so it saves water. Organically farmed soil is rich in nutrients and retains more water. Unfortunately, organic farmers receive few subsidies. This is because most governments support the chemical industry that supplies chemical fertilizers to conventional farming. Organic foods are not subjected to irradiation, chemical additives or industrial solvents.

Does all of this make a difference? Promoters of conventional factory farming will cite studies that include macronutrients and a limited selection of micronutrients and conclude that organic foods are no different from conventionally farmed foods. Newer studies that include a full spectrum of micronutrients, show that some organic foods do have an advantage. The problem with only looking at nutrients, is that it does not take into account the total chemical and pesticide loading. Each of the major industries such as the meat producers, dairy producers and processed food producers, claim that their foods do not cause health problems if eaten in reasonable amounts. Yet these foods combined, clearly cause disease and poor health.

I say go organic where possible. If it is too expensive, pick which foods benefit most from buying organic. This is covered in the section "Food toxins" later in this chapter. In the United States, organic labeling on foods is controlled by the National Organic Program that is part of the USDA and the regulations change from time to time, so it is a good idea to check the latest rules as to what organic actually means. At the time this book was published organic had the following meaning:

- If labeled "100% organic" the food must contain only organically produced ingredients.
- If labeled "Organic" the food must contain 95% organically produced ingredients.
- If labeled "Made with organic ingredients" the food must contain at least 70% organically produced ingredients.

Keep your guard up, because there is some conventionally farmed food being sold as organic by unscrupulous sellers. Unless you are buying food directly from a farm or CSA, you can't be 100% sure that you are getting organic food. There are no quick tests to verify that food is really organic. The penalties for selling conventional foods as organic, are not severe enough to discourage this practice and enforcement is minimal or nonexistent in many areas. The food industry has a track record of mislabeling food products. For example, recent DNA testing of fish has revealed that some species such as tuna and red snapper are mislabeled 57% to 80% of the time! This tells us that if there is an economic incentive and a means to get away with it, some suppliers will engage in deceptive practices.

Cage free & Free range

In the United States and many other countries the terms "cage free" and "free range" are marketing terms and have no official meaning beyond that the animal has to have been let outside at some point in its life! Furthermore there is no monitoring or enforcement. In the European Union, there are regulations defining what free range means including stipulations for time outside, type of ground cover, how many animals per unit of land area, etc.

Wild

Wild vegetables and fruit are very nutritious. If you are going to forage for wild varieties yourself, make sure to get a good book on the subject and also go with someone experienced. Use caution, some wild varieties of edible plants are similar to species that are poisonous and can be easily mistaken. If you are foraging for wild food anywhere close to human activity, make sure to be aware of pesticide spraying in the area. Strong pesticides are sometimes used in areas not used for domestic food production.

What about "health food" or lightly processed food?

This is a question that gets asked a lot, mainly in regard to supposedly "healthy" processed food or lightly processed foods such as granola, whole wheat bread, oat bran muffins, orange juice, etc. The best answer is to not eat processed food. On a practical level most people do eat some of these foods, so the best practical answer is to eat the minimum amount possible and pick the ones with the least amount of processing.

It is also important to make the distinction between processed food and whole food that has some amount of processing done to it. An example of this is brown rice compared to white rice. Brown rice has been de-husked, but is otherwise a whole food. White rice on the other hand has been overly processed, removing most of the nutrients. In many cases whole foods go through a limited amount of processing such as de-husking and washing, which is OK. The problem is when the processing destroys the nutritional value of the food or changes the energy density.

Most stores sell food that is marketed as "whole", "whole grain", "healthy", "natural", "old fashioned", "country", "pure", "original", "nutritious", etc. Unfortunately, most of the time these are empty marketing words and the foods have similar ingredients to other processed foods. If the information in chapter two was not enough to make you stop eating processed foods altogether, read a book called "Pandora's Lunch Box: How processed food took over the American meal" by Melanie Warner. This book is dedicated to examining processed foods and gives a shocking look at the chemicals that are used to make processed foods.

If you are looking at food and trying to determine if it is healthy, look at the list of ingredients. If the list of ingredients is short and simple, and you recognize everything, and there are no bad ingredients, then this is a minimally processed food. An example is old fashioned peanut butter. The ingredient list reads; peanuts, salt. This is a minimally processed food because the peanuts have been put through a grinder and a little salt was added, but in this case there was not enough processing to nutritionally damage the peanuts or change the energy density. Nothing was added or removed (except for the small amount of salt).

What about soda?

Most types of popularly available soda, both regular or diet are loaded with artificial chemicals and sweeteners and should be avoided, but It really depends on what type of soda and what is in it. For example, lets look at diet citrus soda with an ingredient list that reads; filtered water, carbon dioxide, citric acid, aspartame. The undesirable ingredients are citric acid and aspartame. Citric acid is undesirable in this case because it is chemically refined and concentrated and not in its natural form. We can get plenty of citric acid from oranges and other natural sources, we don't need processed citric acid from a factory. Aspartame is a chemical based artificial sweetener and of course should be avoided. An acceptable alternative to diet citrus soda is club soda (carbonated water) with a squirt of lemon.

Most club soda is just water and carbon dioxide. Squeezed lemon or orange could be added. In this case the only issue could be trace chemicals such as the mold release agents used in the manufacturing of the plastic bottle if the club soda was purchased in a plastic bottle. This could be avoided by making your own carbonated water. There are machines you can buy to do this.

Bread and pasta

Some people are able to exclude processed food from their diet completely. That means eliminating all breads and pasta. Most people find it enough to limit eating bread and pasta to once or twice a week. Eating bread and pasta made from whole grains with the least amount of processed ingredients also helps. For pasta, there are several brands made from whole grains that are sold in most grocery stores.

For breads, this usually means baking at home. Very few commercial bakeries make anything that would remotely qualify as lightly processed bread. Many brands of bread are marketed as being whole and lightly processed, but don't live up to the marketing. There is no regulation for this, they can say one thing and do another and most people don't know the difference anyway, they are selling the illusion of healthy bread.

Whole grain old world bread is nothing like the modern commercial bread sold in stores. If you are looking for a healthy replacement to the modern breads you are familiar with, there is none. Modern baked goods are processed foods and there is no way to make them into a whole food. If you want to make old world whole grain bread yourself, sources of organic stone ground flour are covered in chapter six.

Coatings, treatments and wax

Some fruit and vegetables are coated with chemicals or wax by suppliers. This is done to inhibit rotting and oxidation or for aesthetic reasons. Special soaps and rinses are sold for this, but are generally no better than washing with regular soap and water. The best solution is to buy fruit and vegetables that have not been coated or sprayed in the first place. As stated earlier, organic food generally does not look pristine and shiny, but that is a good thing because waxes and chemicals have not been applied.

Food Toxins

Everyday you can read about some new toxin in the food supply. It is easy to get fed up and quit worrying about it altogether, except that food toxins are a serious threat to your health. Fortunately, there is good game plan to deal with this:

Step one - The whole food diet. By eating a whole food diet you will decrease your intake of food toxins by a large amount compared to the standard American diet. Even if you eat factory farmed vegetables and fruits, you will still be making a major improvement by eliminating the dairy and processed foods and cutting down or eliminating meat.

Step two - Do your research. A good place to start is www.ewg.org the web site for the Environmental Working Group, a non profit organization that puts out the "Shoppers Guide to Pestisides in Produce". They also publish the "Clean Fifteen" and the "Dirty Dozen" lists. The data comes from tests done by the US Environmental Protection Agency. The data is available directly from the EPA, but it is in a format that makes it difficult to understand. This causes it to be inaccessible to the average person who just wants to know which foods are safe and which foods are a health hazard. Shame on the EPA.

Step three - Buy organic foods where needed. Organic foods have lower toxins. In a perfect world, if cost was not an issue, we should buy all organic foods, because organic foods have benefits way beyond lower toxins, such as protecting the environment and the health of farmers.

Step four - Buy from food co-ops and community supported agriculture (CSA). These farms grow organic foods locally and you buy directly from the farm, taking out the middle men. Some CSA's allow participation where you can work on the farm and help out. This is not the same as a farmers market. We will go into CSA's more in chapter six.

Step five - Grow your own. You can grow food even in an apartment! Growing your own food is a great way to know exactly what you are getting. It also can save a lot of money and will save you time going to the store.

Step six - Have a voice. Demand improvements. Demand transparency. Don't just take being subjected to dangerous food toxins lying down. Voice your concern. Try to do something about it.

Protecting yourself from food toxins is an ongoing process and requires constant vigilance.

6 - Shopping & Grocery Lists

In this chapter we will cover grocery lists and talk about shopping for whole foods from grocery stores, farmers markets, CSA's (Community Supported Agriculture) and online.

Master list of whole foods

The master list below has most common whole foods. We will use this master list to make our grocery lists. The foods are listed according to the section of a grocery store where they are normally found and not by the actual classification, for example a tomato is actually a fruit, but is classified as a vegetable in most grocery stores.

There are some locally grown varieties of food that are not on the master list. For example, in Asia there are different varieties of pears with different names. Generally they have similar nutritional value and can be substituted. In many countries there are different names for the same species. For example, chickpeas are also called garbanzo beans or channa.

Fresh Vegetables:

- Leaf Vegetables - Collard greens, Kale, Mustard greens, Turnip greens, Watercress, Spinach, Swiss chard, Bok choy, Arugula, Cilantro, Parsley, Cabbage, Brussels sprouts, Romaine lettuce, Napa Cabbage, Broccoli, Cauliflower, Iceberg lettuce, etc.

- Alliums - Yellow onion, Red onion, Garlic, Leek, Chive, Shallot, Scallion (green onion), Other onions, etc.

- Peppers - Red bell pepper, Green bell pepper, Chili pepper, etc.

- Tomato - Tomatoes of all types.

- Root Vegetables - Carrot, Beet, Turnip, Rutabaga, Radish, Parsnip, Sunroot, etc.

- Mushrooms - Shiitake, Portobello, Cremini, White, Brown, Oyster, etc.

- Tubers - Yam, Potato, Sweet potato, Yuca root, Taro, etc.

- Squashes - Pumpkin, Cucumber, Zucchini, Yellow Squash, Eggplant, Acorn squash, etc.

- Stalks & Shoots - Asparagus, Celery, Rhubarb, Bamboo, wheatgrass, etc.

- Legumes - Green beans, Snap peas, Snow peas, Edamame, Soy bean sprouts, Mung bean sprouts, etc.

- Other Vegetables - Okra, Artichoke, Sunchoke, etc.

- Herbs & Spices - Mint, Dill, Oregano, Turmeric, Sage, Fennel, Rosemary, Basil, Tea Leaf, Thyme, Lavender, Coriander, Paprika, Ginger, etc

- Wild Plants & Weeds - Purslane, Dandelion, Amaranth, Chickweed, Tart greens, Wintercress, Garlic mustard, etc.

Fresh Fruit & Berries:

- Tropical Fruit - Avocado, Pineapple, Banana, Plantain, Mango, Guava, Coconut, Passion fruit, Papayas, Breadfruit, Jackfruit, etc.

- Citrus Fruit - Orange, Grapefruit, Lemon, lime, etc.

- Tree Fruit - Apple, Pear, Apricot, Cherry, Peach, Plum, Rose Hip, Nectarine, Persimmon, Tamarind, etc.

- Berries - Blackberry, Blueberry, Boysenberry, Cranberry, Huckleberry, Raspberry, Mulberry, Strawberry, etc.

- Vine Fruit - Grape, Kiwi, Raisin, Currant, etc.

- Mediterranean Fruit - Date, Fig, Pomegranate, etc.

- Melons - Watermelon, Cantaloupe, Casaba, Winter melon, Honeydew, etc.

Frozen Food:

- Leaf Vegetables - Collard greens, Kale, Mustard greens, Turnip greens, Spinach, Brussels sprouts, Broccoli, Cauliflower, etc.

- Berries - Blackberry, Blueberry, Boysenberry, Cranberry, Huckleberry, Raspberry, Mulberry, Strawberry, Mixed frozen berries, etc.

- Tropical Fruit - Pineapple, Mango, Passion fruit, Papaya, Mixed frozen tropical fruit, etc.

- Legumes - Lima bean, Green pea, Edamame, Fava bean, Green bean, Snap pea, Snow pea, Black eyed peas, etc.

- Assorted Vegetables - Stir fry mix, Okra, Mixed vegetables, etc.

- Frozen Juice (for use as a sweetener) - Orange, Grape, Cranberry, etc.

Dried Food:

- Legumes - Lentil (green, red, yellow), Lima bean, Chickpea, Desi chickpea, Pinto bean, Black bean, Green split peas, Soy bean, Kidney bean, Black eyed pea, Fava bean, Snap pea, Snow pea, Mung bean, Mayocoba beans, etc.

- Seeds- Flax seed (ground), Sesame, Hemp seed, Chia, Sunflower seeds, Pumpkin seeds, etc.

- Nuts - Walnut, Hazelnut, Peanut, Almond, Brazil nut, Pecan, Cashew, etc.

- Grains - Brown rice, Parboiled rice, Oatmeal, Wheat berries, Barley, Corn, Millet, Rye, Quinoa, Sorghum (Milo), Buckwheat, bulgur wheat, spelt, etc.

- Sea Vegetables - Wakame, Kombu, Nori, etc.

- Mushrooms - Shiitake, Portobello, Cremini, White, Brown, Oyster, etc.
- Flour - Stone ground whole grain flour; Wheat, Buckwheat, Spelt, Sorghum, Corn, Oat, Chickpea, Amaranth, 10 grain, masa harina (hominy), etc.

Cans, Bottles & Cartons:

- Canned - Tomato Sauce, Tomato Paste, DIced tomato, Curry paste, Chili pepper paste, etc.
- Bottles (and Jars) - White Vinegar, Apple cider vinegar, Peanut butter, Almond butter, Applesauce, Molasses, etc.
- Cartons - Organic Tofu, Tempeh, Vegetable stock, etc.

Dry Spices & Seasonings:

- Herbs and Spices - Thyme, Cumin seed, Ceylon cinnamon, Coriander seed, Oregano, Turmeric, Fennel seed, Curry powder, Paprika, Black Peppercorns (use with a pepper mill), Red pepper flakes, Chili pepper, Black pepper.
- Buy when needed Herbs and Spices - Basil, Sage, Mint, Dill, Rosemary, Tea Leaf, Lavender, Ginger, Garlic powder, Allspice, Nutmeg, Ground cloves, Jalapeno pepper, Cayenne pepper, Parsley, Ground Onion, Alum, Bay leaves, Caraway seed, Mustard seed, Sesame seed, Saffron, Poppy seed, Anise seed, Arrowroot, ground onion, Miso power.
- Seasonings - Italian seasoning, Season-All, Chili mix, Taco seasoning, Mrs Dash, Lemon pepper, Garlic pepper, etc.
- Salt - Table salt (iodized), Sea salt (iodized).

Miscellaneous items:

- Vitamin B12
- Vitamin D3
- Red Star nutritional yeast. This is an alternative source of vitamin B12

International section:

- Indian - Chickpeas, Desi chickpeas, Lentils, Turmeric powder, Curry, Coriander powder, Cumin seed, etc.
- Asian - Soy sauce, Sriracha sauce, Garlic sauce, Spices, Mustard sauce, Wakame, Kombu, Nori, Dried Mushrooms, Dried fish, Canned oysters, etc.
- Hispanic - Chile peppers, Salsa, Refried beans, Black beans, Hot sauces, Parboiled rice, etc.
- Mediterranean - Tahini, Hummus, Couscous, Tabbouleh, Toum, Chickpeas, Desi chickpeas, Lentils, etc.

Drinks:

- Tea (dry in tea bags) - Green tea, Black tea, Earl Gray, Green tea with ginger, etc.
- Club soda (carbonated water).

Animal Based Foods:

- Meat - Chicken, Turkey, Beef, Pork, Bison, Venison, Emu, Ostrich, etc.
- Fish - Salmon, Tilapia, Carp, Catfish, Tuna, Sardines, Sturgeon, Halibut, Cod, Mackerel, etc.
- Seafood - Clams, Oysters, Mussels, Scallops, Octopus, Squid, Snails, Abalone, Cuttlefish, Crab, Shrimp, Prawns, Crayfish, etc.
- Eggs

Example grocery lists

In this section we will present an example grocery list made using foods from the master list.

Basic low cost grocery list:

- Fresh Vegetables - Kale, Cabbage, Broccoli, Yellow onion, Mushrooms, Sweet potato, Eggplant, Zucchini.
- Fresh Fruit & Berries - Avocado, Pineapple, Banana, Grapefruit, Pear, Blueberry.
- Frozen Food - Collard greens, Spinach, Brussels sprouts, Mixed frozen berries, Lima beans.
- Frozen Juice (for use as a sweetener) - Orange, Grape.
- Dried Food - Lentil, Chickpea, Black bean, Green split peas, Flax seed (ground), Brown rice, Oatmeal, Stone ground 10 grain flour.
- Cans, Bottles & Cartons - Tomato Paste, Tomato sauce, Organic Tofu, Tempeh, Vegetable stock.
- Herbs and Spices - Thyme, Cumin seed, Ceylon cinnamon, Coriander seed, Oregano, Fennel seed, Curry powder, Paprika, Black Peppercorns (use with a pepper mill), Red pepper flakes, Chili pepper, Black pepper.
- Seasonings - Italian seasoning, Season-All, Taco seasoning, Mrs Dash.
- Salt - Table salt (iodized).
- Miscellaneous items - Vitamin B12, Vitamin D3.
- Drinks - Green tea, Black tea, club soda.
- Animal Based Foods: Sardines (canned).

Explanation for basic low cost list:

This is a good basic list to start, if you are new to a whole food diet. The foods on the list are available in most grocery stores. After you are familiar with the items on the list, you can start branching out and trying new foods that you have not eaten before. You don't need to buy all the items at one time. All of the frozen, dry and canned items can be purchased on a monthly or bi-monthly basis if you prefer, but the fresh vegetables and fruit should be replenished in smaller amounts, two or three times a week. To reduce your trips to the store, you can buy fresh vegetables and fruit and freeze them.

In most areas of the United States, it should be possible to feed one person using the items on this list for under $200 per month. This completely dispels the myth that a whole food diet is expensive. Most people eating an American diet spend more than $200 on fast food and eating out.

Your grocery list

There are two ways to make your grocery list, meals first or foods first:

Meals first - After you read through chapters seven, eight and nine, make a list of the meals you want to prepare and add the required foods to your grocery list. Make a note of the quantity of each food that is needed, so you will know how much to buy.

Foods first - Start by looking at the master list and adding an item or two from each category, until you have a nice looking selection of foods in your grocery list. You can then adapt your meals and recipes to work with the foods that you have purchased. Another idea is to start with the basic low cost list and just add or remove items to make it your own.

Rotation list

Each food has different types of nutrients and eating a broad variety insures that you will have the broadest selection of nutrients possible. Over time, you should try to eat most of the foods on the master list, at least every once in a while. To do this, make a copy of the master list. Each time you go shopping, buy one or two foods from the list that you don't normally buy. As you buy a food, cross it off the list. When all foods are crossed off, make a new copy of the master list and start over again. This is your rotation list.

Fresh, frozen, dried or canned?

Fresh vegetables - Fresh should be your first choice when available. Check various stores to find the best deals. When you find a good deal, buy more than you need and freeze some. It is important to find reasonably priced vegetables, because you should eat lots of them. If they are too expensive or there is no convenient source (like during the winter season), you should buy them frozen. The frozen section will not have as large a selection, but frozen vegetables will hold you over until fresh vegetables are available at a reasonable cost.

In most areas you can buy the fresh leafy green vegetables like kale, collard greens and mustard greens in one or two pound bags, pre-cut and pre-washed. If you can't find them, ask. If they don't have them, find a store that does.

Fresh fruit - Try eating a piece before you buy! You can do this by buying one piece or sometimes the grocer will allow you to try a piece. With many types of fruit and vegetables, this is the only way to be sure of what you are getting and to avoid force ripened or rotting fruit.

Frozen vegetables and fruit - Frozen vegetables and fruit usually do not taste quite as good as fresh, but they hold their nutritional value quite well. Frozen food lasts a long time and is there when you need it.

Dried food - Dried food such as legumes and grains have a long shelf life between 6 months to a year or more. Dried food usually comes in plastic bags or is stocked in the bulk food section. Most dried legumes can be sprouted. Once sprouted, they become a fresh food, this takes a couple days.

Flour - There are several companies that specialized in organic stone ground whole grain flours with no added preservatives or other unwanted ingredients. Bob's Red Mill products are now available in most grocery stores. Great River Organic Milling and Palouse Brand are two others. Also check out alternative flours such as almond flour. On-line sellers such as Amazon.com and eBay carry many brands of whole grain flours and healthy baking supplies.

Canned & Bottled Food - The advantage of canned and bottled food is the long shelf life. Canned and bottled food does not taste as good as fresh or frozen food. Watch the ingredient list closely, most canned and bottled foods have unwanted additives and large amounts of salt. Wikipedia is a good source of information about food ingredients. If you are at the store and have a smartphone, you can look up ingredients that look strange or dangerous before you buy something.

Grocery stores

There are some stores that take an interest in the health of their customers and the environment. Stores that care, take steps to do some or all of the following:

- Eliminate harmful ingredients in their products such as; hydrogenated oils, artificial flavors, artificial colors, sweeteners, chemical preservatives, hormones, antibiotics, fungicides, etc.

- Complete and honest disclosure of ingredients.

- Promote organic foods and humanely produced animal products.

- Promote sustainably produced products and practices.

- Supply chain transparency, such as what farm the product came and how the farm is run.

Listed below are some examples of stores that address one or more of the issues on the above list. This is not an exhaustive list, just a profile of some positive things that a few stores are doing. If you can find one of these stores in your area, it is worth checking out, even if it means traveling a distance. If none of these stores are close by, ask around to find similar stores that are in your area.

Whole Foods Market - 387 stores in the US, Canada and UK. They have an informative rating system for their meat, fish and seafood products. The company website has a lot of nutritional and food preparation information. Wikipedia has an informative page on Whole Foods Market.

Trader Joe's - 418 stores in the US. Owned by German company Aldi Nord. Trader Joe's labeled products (sold under the Trader Joe's brand name) feature non-GMO ingredients and the elimination of many unwanted ingredients and preservatives. The company website has recipes and food preparation information.

Harris Teeter - 231 stores in the US, owned by Kroger as of 2014. Harris Teeter has a healthy eating program and scores well on seafood sustainability rankings. They sell bulk foods. Fresh foods can be ordered online and then picked up at store locations.

Safeway - 1335 stores in the US, merged with A&P in July 2014. For all outward appearances Safeway looks like just another grocer, but under the surface something is brewing! They have consistently scored above other major grocery store chains in sustainability areas such as transparency, policy and supplier involvement. They are increasing the amount of organic products in their stores and reducing retail prices for organics. It remains to be seen if the merger with A&P will derail their progress.

Farmers markets

Farmers markets were widespread many years ago and were a place where farmers came to sell their crops to the townspeople. Recently there has been a renewed interest in the concept of farmers markets and many entrepreneurs have sprung up to service this market. Some of these entrepreneurs are real farmers, others are simply retailers that get product from normal distribution channels and use farmers markets as a sales channel. There are also middlemen dumping substandard products through farmers markets. There is little or no regulation of farmers markets in most areas and many vendors are here today, gone tomorrow.

Keep you eyes open and ask questions. Your local farmers market could be a real gem, or it could be a fake. In my experience less than half of farmers markets are the real thing. Look at the food closely, does it look like small farm grown organic food or does it look like the same polished and waxed food you see at the local grocery store, but at a higher price. Ask if you can go visit the farm, and then really do it.

Community supported agriculture (CSA)

In many areas a CSA may be your best source for high quality produce at a reasonable cost. Community supported agriculture (CSA) is also called community shared agriculture. Basically most CSA's are local organic farms who sell a subscription or membership by the year or by the month. The customer commits to a monthly or yearly fee and in return, the farm makes available allotments of fresh vegetables and other foods on a bi-weekly basis (or other schedule) during the growing season. Some CSA's have trucks to deliver the food to customers, others require the customers to pick up the food from the farm or a distribution point. Many CSA's have programs to let the customers help out with planting, maintenance and harvesting. There are many types of CSA's including member owned, farmer owned, member managed, etc. Wikipedia is a good place to start researching about CSA's, search for "community supported agriculture".

Shopping online

In many areas it may be difficult to find high quality organic food. Shopping online is a way to get many types of foods without traveling long distances or doing a lot of unnecessary running around. Amazon.com sells a large amount of organic food and has good customer service and good prices. There are many other online stores, also don't forget eBay. Online sellers are a great source for nuts, seeds, stone ground whole grain flour, raisins, spices, seasonings, herbs, etc. Some online sellers now sell produce and fruit, in some areas it is possible to do your grocery shopping online.

Shopping

If you have your grocery list and your rotation list in hand, you are ready to go shopping.

Shop often - The modern idea of grocery shopping in which you go to the grocery store and buy enough food for one or two weeks works with a processed food diet, but is not suitable for a whole food diet, because fresh whole foods are perishable. A good idea is to go major shopping once every week or two and buy the full shopping list including frozen, dry and canned foods. Twice or three times a week, go minor shopping for perishable foods. An alternative is to freeze the fresh food, in this case it is possible to shop once or twice a month, if getting to the grocery store is problematic.

Shop at several stores - Most people shop mainly at one grocery store. With a whole food diet this will either end up costing too much or will limit your selection of food. It helps to shop at more than one store to take advantage of specials. Some stores have a better selection of fresh food than other stores. Shopping at several stores sounds time consuming, but it really is not.

The international section - In the International food section of most stores, you will find many ingredients that are great for whole food diets at very good prices. Some of the seasonings in the international section are available in large packages, for a fraction of the cost of similar seasonings in the regular seasoning section.

The bulk food section - Most grocery stores now have a bulk food section. Bulk food has no packaging and is sold from large bins. Bulk food is dried, and mostly consists of grains, legumes and nuts. Prices for bulk food is normally less than packaged food, and a larger selection is available. For example, wheat berries are available in most bulk food sections, but are not normally available as a packaged product. Herbs and spices are available in most bulk food sections at much lower prices.

Vigilance while shopping

To maintain a good diet you must continually make decisions about what you should buy and what you should eat. New information is constantly being discovered. This is an ongoing process. The profit motive is always there in the food industry, this is human nature. It should also be human nature to continually protect ourselves and be vigilant. Don't get complacent! Modifications and ingredient substitutions are common as suppliers try to maximize profits. This may be done slowly, so that customers won't notice the difference. The foods you evaluated and liked last year, can become something totally different this year. Watch for differences in the appearance, taste or texture of the foods that you buy.

7 - Cooking & Preparation

This chapter starts with cooking and cooking equipment. Later in the chapter, cooking instructions for many types of food are covered along with baking, sprouting and fermentation.

About cooking

Reasons to cook:

- Soften tough food so that it can be eaten (rice or beans).
- Remove naturally occurring bitterness (some greens).
- Kill harmful bacteria (meat).
- Neutralize naturally occurring toxins (kidney beans).
- Help remove pesticides (commercially grown food).

Nutritional loss in cooking - Lightly cooking causes minimal nutritional loss. For most foods the loss of vitamins and other nutrients is about 10-30%, depending on the food and the cooking time. Some foods such as carrots and other root vegetables, benefit from cooking and have an increase in nutrients. Overall the nutrient loss from cooking is not a significant concern. The nutritional analysis software and food composition databases covered in chapter eleven can be used to compare cooked and uncooked foods on an individual nutrient level.

Cooking commercially grown food - The case for lightly cooking commercially grown foods is strong, because commercially grown foods can be grown with substandard fertilizers such as biosolids (sewage sludge), chemical fertilizers and chemical pesticides. Cooking will kill harmful bacteria and help to neutralize some of these threats. Because there is little transparency or disclosure in the United States, you have no idea what fertilizers and pesticides have been used with conventional crops.

Cooking organically grown food - The case for cooking organic food is not as strong, because organic food is free from most chemicals and pesticides. When you eat raw food, it is much better to go with organic food, home grown food, or food from a CSA or local farm. As we talked about in chapter three, if you are new to a whole food diet, don't start out with huge salads or plates of raw vegetables, instead lightly cook most of your vegetables and gradually increase the amount of raw vegetables to give your digestive system time to build up the needed bacteria.

Cook times and temperatures

To preserve the nutritional value and character of the food, use the minimum amount of cooking time that is needed to achieve the goals of cooking. Most food should require a substantial amount of chewing. Chewing causes the release of saliva that is a necessary part of the digestive process. In the American diet, there is little or no thought given to preserving the nutritional value or character of the food and most vegetables are cooked into a non-nutritional mush, so that little or no chewing is required.

Achieving the correct cooking time is often a matter of trial and error, it helps to occasionally test food while it is cooking to see if it is cooked enough. This is particularly helpful if you are cooking varieties of food that you have never cooked before. Leaf vegetables should be cooked just enough to kill bacteria and to soften them up just a little, if they are tough. For kale, it is enough to boil it for a few minutes. Collard greens need to be cooked a little longer, until they are tender enough to eat.

Small frozen foods like lima beans and green peas can be cooked without thawing, but it is best to thaw larger frozen foods like Brussels sprouts. If you are in a hurry you can use a sink full of hot water to rapidly thaw frozen food.

Cooking and food safety

For some foods there is a mandatory minimum cooking temperature and time that is needed to neutralize naturally occurring toxins and bacteria such as E.coli, salmonella, oxalic acid and phytohaemagglutinin. An example of these foods are meat, fish, seafood, eggs, most legumes and some vegetables. Achieving the correct cooking time and temperature is very important, because when properly cooked these foods are safe, but if they are not cooked correctly they can be toxic. If you are cooking a new variety of food that you are not familiar with, it is a good idea to look it up or ask someone who knows, to make sure that you know the special cooking requirements relating to safety and toxins.

Cooking methods

There are many cooking methods. We will go over the ones that lend themselves to cooking with whole foods and point out the ones to avoid because they are bad for nutrition or health.

Blanching and parboiling - You can think of blanching as "boil, pour and cool". In blanching a pot of water is brought to a brisk boil and food is added for a brief time lasting from a few seconds to several minutes, depending on the food being cooked. Next, the food is removed from the water or the water is poured out. Cold water is used to rapidly cool the food and stop the food from cooking. You can think of parboiling as "boil and pour". It is the same as blanching, except the last step of cooling the food with cold water is not done, the food is allowed to cool on it's own after the boiling water is poured out.

Blanching and parboiling are great methods for cooking whole foods, because the rapidly boiling water is hot enough to kill bacteria and remove many types of toxins and pesticides from the surface of food. With biosolids being increasingly used as fertilizer, the danger of bacteria from conventionally grown crops is very real and blanching or parboiling addresses this issue. If short cooking times are used, the nutritional integrity of food is not damaged. Another advantage of blanching and parboiling is that they are fast.

Blanching and parboiling are the best methods to cook many types of vegetables such as collard greens, kale, spinach and similar green leafy vegetables. When organic vegetables are cooked, after parboiling, the water that is drained can be used as a stock for other cooking. With conventionally farmed vegetables this is not advisable, because the water may contain pesticides, chemical fertilizer residue or conditioning sprays from the vegetables being cooked.

Boiling and simmering - Food is boiled or simmered in water or some other liquid comprised mostly of water such as broth or vegetable stock. Boiling occurs at 212 degrees fahrenheit (100 centigrade). At this temperature large bubbles will form briskly. Simmering is done by briefly heating the food to a brisk boil and then reducing the temperature slightly, until the food is cooking at just under a boiling temperature (180 to 200 degrees). At this temperature small bubbles will form. Boiling and simmering are the primary methods used to cook legumes and grains such as beans and rice.

Steaming - Steaming can be done with a pot of boiling water and a perforated container to hold the food above the boiling water. Special steaming pots are made for this purpose. Steaming has the advantage of removing less of the nutrients than other methods of cooking, because there is no direct contact with the water to wash away the nutrients. However, steaming is less effective at removing pesticides and toxins from the food. This makes steaming a good choice for organic vegetables, blanching or parboiling may be a better choice for conventionally grown crops. Steaming works better for foods that allow the steam to move through them such as broccoli and Brussels sprouts, steaming may not work well for foods that block the circulation of steam such as collard greens or kale.

Sauteing, frying and stir frying - These methods are traditionally done in a pan with oil, but can be done at a slightly lower temperature with no oil or a greatly reduced amount of oil for healthier cooking. As a substitute for oil, vegetable stock can be used with a few drops of oil and possibly some vinegar or cooking wine. Other seasonings and spices can be added.

Baking - Baking is a dry cooking method done in an oven. Baking is great for potatoes, yams, casserole, squash, meats, bread, etc.

Pressure cooking - In pressure cooking, food is cooked under steam pressure. Pressure cooking requires a special pot called a pressure cooker. The advantage is that food cooks faster under pressure and requires less water and energy. While boiling kills most microorganisms, pressure cooking offers almost complete sterilization. A pressure cooker can be used as a sterilizer for baby items and other items.

Deep frying - Deep frying should be avoided, because it is done in oil, and because it is done at high temperatures that nutritionally damage food and cause the formation of toxic and carcinogenic chemicals such as acrylamide.

Grilling, roasting, broiling, barbecuing and smoking - These cooking methods should be avoided, because they are done at high temperatures or involve direct contact with fire and combustion byproducts that cause the formation of toxic and carcinogenic chemicals such as acrylamide, furan, tar, soot, etc.

Slow cooking - Slow cooking should be avoided, because it is done over long time periods that destroy the nutritional value of food.

Cookware

Cooking with whole foods requires a minimum amount of inexpensive cookware. Simple stainless steel pots, pans and cookware are the best, because they are more durable. Check the pricing and reviews online before buying cookware and equipment. Also check out your local restaurant supply store for heavy duty cookware that is built to last, this may cost more but in the long run you will save money.

Pots & pans - You don't need the heavy and expensive pots and pans with multilayer copper clad bottoms, in fact some of my favorite pots are lighter single or double layer stainless steel types, because they are much easier to handle and to pour. A pot of boiling water is already heavy enough, but when the empty pot weighs a lot by itself, it is harder to handle. There is little advantage in the way that heavy multilayer pots heat, in fact it takes longer to get a heavy pot to heat up, because of the thermal mass of the metal. Avoid teflon or other coated pots and pans for health reasons and because they don't last long. Stainless steel pots and pans can last for more than 50 years.

A 2 or 3 quart pot is the perfect size for cooking 16 ounce packages of dried legumes, making rice, soup and many other tasks. Use a 3 or 4 quart pot if you want to add more ingredients or for combinations such as rice and beans. An 8 quart stock pot is ideal for cooking one or two pounds of fresh greens at a time, this is about right if you are cooking for two people. Some stock pots come with a steaming basket. For a family of three or four you may want a 12 or 16 quart stock pot. For one or two people use a 12 inch stainless steel fry pan. If you have a big family you may need a larger one. Some people prefer a cast iron skillet.

Don't forget the lids! It takes much longer to heat a pot without a lid, because the exchange of air in the pot slows the heating. After the pot is heated, it takes a lower setting for a covered pot to maintain a simmering temperature. Glass lids look nice, but they condensate, you can't see what is going on inside the pot. For this reason you may want to save your money and get stainless steel lids that last forever.

Wok - A wok is a large curved pan that is used for stir frying. The advantage of a wok is that the the liquid rolls down to the lowest point in the center of the wok, this is the point that receives the most heat from the burner. This allows a wok to cook at higher temperatures without burning.

Baking pans - Get a few sizes. If you can get the glass or stainless steel pans that come with covers they are handy, you can use them to store and refrigerate the food without transferring it. Make sure that glass pans are made from pyrex or some other type of oven safe high temperature glass.

Salad bowls - Stainless steel salad bowls are inexpensive and will last a lifetime.

Sealable glass or plastic containers - A must for storing extra food for the next meal.

Sprouter - There are many types of sprouting jars and sprouting racks available that make sprouting easier.

Cooking utensils

Knives - You don't need a large set of knifes, an 8 inch chefs knife and an 8 inch bread knife are a good first purchase. These can be relatively inexpensive stainless steel. My favorites are the Dexter-Russell Sani-safe knives with the white handles, but even the Farberware knives sold at Walmart work fine. I use a bread knife with the serrated edge for many types of food, because it will slice through food that other types of knives will crush and make a mess out of. It is also great for cutting large fruit such as watermelon.

Hand-held vegetable peelers - There are two types of hand held peelers, the straight peeler and the julienne peeler. The straight peeler is good for removing the peel from fruit and vegetables, it can even handle thick peels like cassava. The julienne peeler is used for thinly slicing vegetables like carrots and cucumbers.

Mixing spoons, Spatula, Grater, Measuring cups, Measuring spoons, Strainer or colander - My preference again is stainless steel, they last longer and are easier to clean. For sure you should get a stainless steel turner (spatula) with a thin and flat blade. The thin blade can slide under the food without smushing it and making a mess, this is what professional chefs use.

Large 4 cup glass measuring cup - For measuring larger quantities and mixing stuff.

Mortar and pestle - For crushing seeds and smashing garlic.

Tea infuser - There are many types of tea infusers, but they all hold loose tea leaves so that they can be immersed in boiling water to make tea. Most infusers consist of a stainless steel mesh ball that opens like a clamshell to insert the tea. Most have a handle or a chain to lower the ball into the boiling water.

Machines

Blender - For making smoothies and blending food. Don't get a poorly made inexpensive model. I recommend the KitchenAid 5 speed blenders that sell for about $90 to $120 or more, depending on the color (many colors are available). This blender has a heavy and strong motor, whereas most blenders have a heavy weighted base, with a wimpy motor that will soon smell like burnt wiring if you do any serious blending. Ignore the wattage rating of blenders. The watts rating only tells you how much power the blender uses, not how powerful the motor is. Some blenders use most of their power to heat up the room and make noise instead of actually blending food. The best way to test a blender is making hummus. Thick hummus will make most blenders die within minutes. Of course be sure to check the online reviews.

Immersion blender - Also called a hand blender. They make small ones and larger models that are very powerful. The advantage is that you blend the food in any stainless steel cooking pot, just stick the blender in when you want to blend. Larger models can blend huge stock pots of food quickly. You can then cook the food right in the same pot, no extra washing! This is what they use in commercial kitchens, they don't use the home type blenders. Go online and read the reviews before buying one of these.

Spiralizer - A spiralizer (spiral vegetable slicer) is an inexpensive hand powered device for quickly cutting vegetables into strands. The device has a hand crank that is used to rotate the vegetable against some cutting blades. The advantage of a spiralizer over a food processor (for some types of cutting), is easy setup and cleaning and there is no container to limit how much you cut at one time. Search for "spiralizer" on Amazon.com to see the types that are available and get an idea of features and prices.

Food processor - Great for shredding and chopping food, a food processor does not require added water, whereas a blender is usually used when the end result is a liquid. Most food processors have several interchangeable blades for different food types. Do some serious online research before buying a food processor. There are a lot of horrible food processors being sold, some expensive ones that look high tech are no good. Look at the ratings and read comments before you make a decision.

Mixer - Mixers come in hand held types or stand mixers like the popular KitchenAid models that are sold everywhere. Some stand mixers have an attachment point so that other accessories can be mounted. Mixers are mainly used to make dough for baking.

Grinders and mills - If you are making nut butter or grinding grains it is best to use a grinder or a mill. Grinders are better for grinding nut butter and meat, mills are better for grinding dried grains and legumes. Some food processors can make nut butter, but making nut butter will burn out the motor of most food processors. Grinders and mills are powered or hand cranked. The hand cranked versions work well and are quite inexpensive. If you have one of the large KitchenAid stand mixers you can get a grinding attachment for about $50 that uses the powerful motor of the mixer. Good quality stand alone power grinders and mills are more expensive.

Juicers - Juicers are not recommended, because a juicer removes most of the fiber and pulp, leaving a liquid with much of the nutritional content removed and an increased energy level. This is a form of refinement (processing) and is not good from a nutritional standpoint. Instead of juicing, make smoothies!

Ovens & cookers

Microwave oven - Good for warming up food and cooking small amounts of food quickly. Also great for making hot beverages.

Pressure cooker - A pressure cooker is a special heavy-duty pot, with a sealing and locking lid and a pressure regulating valve on the top. Pressure cookers are great for cooking beans in much less time than it takes in a regular pot. Pressure cookers come in regular versions that you heat on the stove and electric versions that plug into the wall. The electric versions have some advanced features (depending on the model) such as a timer. The electric models look similar to a rice cooker.

Rice cooker - Not just for rice, other foods can be cooked in a rice cooker such as millet, quinoa, barley and most other grains. Most models are set-and-forget, so you can do other things while the rice is cooking without the worry of overcooking. This is the real advantage of a rice cooker, actually a rice cooker does nothing else that you can't do yourself with a pot on the stove. With a rice cooker you can start the rice cooking and turn your attention to preparing other foods. By the time you hear the rice cooker beep indicating that it is done, you will probably have just finished cooking the other food. Get an inexpensive and simple rice cooker, there is no advantage to an expensive and complicated rice cooker with silly extra features. It just needs to cook the rice.

Dehydrator - Food dehydrators come in many sizes and have racks or trays that allow for dehydrating more food at one time than can be done in a home oven. Dehydrators use less power than an oven and only get hot enough to dry out the food but not cook it. There are designs on the internet for home made (DIY) dehydrators that use common incandescent light bulbs to generate the heat.

Slow cookers - Slow cookers are not recommended for traditional slow cooking, because slow cookers do not get hot enough to neutralize toxins that are present in some beans such as kidney beans and fava beans. Slow cookers also overcook vegetables and other foods because of the long cooking times. This destroys the nutritional value.

BBQ grills - Barbecue grills are not recommended, because barbecue grills cause the formation of acrylamide and combustion byproducts like soot and tar promote colon cancer and heart disease.

Cooking with little or no oil

Cooking with little or no oil can be handled in various ways. In boiling, parboiling, blanching and steaming there is no need for oil. For baking, frying or stir frying without oil, a slightly lower temperature can be used with water, broth or stock.

When frying or stir frying without oil, always cover your pan. This will reduce the cooking time required, because the food will heat faster. Reduce the temperature a little. Adding ingredients such as pineapple, tomato sauce or concentrated orange juice can add moisture and prevent burning without oil.

Cooking greens and cabbage

Greens and cabbage are best boiled. This includes collard greens, kale, mustard greens, turnip greens, watercress, spinach, cabbage, purslane and amaranth. Frozen greens (except cabbage) can be cooked without thawing, but they will need a longer cooking time. Greens that have similar cooking times can be mixed, such as turnip greens and mustard greens. If you are cooking greens and cabbage, add the greens after the cabbage has been cooking a while, because cabbage needs a longer cooking time.

1. Wash the greens and chop into pieces.
2. Boil enough water to cover the greens. Once the water is briskly boiling, add the greens to the boiling water. Adding the greens after the water is boiling will reduce the cooking time.
3. The length of time to cook will vary from 1 minute to several minutes depending on how you like them cooked, the less time the better from a nutritional perspective. Soft greens such as spinach will need a short cooking time. Tougher greens like collard greens will take up to 10 minutes to cook, especially if parts of the stalks are chopped up with the leaves. Cabbage can take over 15 minutes at a simmer.
4. After the greens are cooked, pour out the water if the greens are not organic (to get rid of any pesticides or contaminates). In the case of organic greens, the water does not need to be fully drained, it can be partially drained and the greens can be seasoned and served in the cooking water.
5. Optionally broth, stock or seasonings can be added.

Cooking broccoli, cauliflower and Brussels sprouts

Broccoli, cauliflower, Brussels sprouts and similar vegetables are best boiled or steamed. If they are frozen let them thaw first. It is best to season after cooking or serve them unseasoned.

- For boiling broccoli and cauliflower the steps are: wash, cut or break into pieces, add to rapidly boiling water, boil from 1 minute to several minutes, pour out the water, set aside to cool.

- For boiling Brussels sprouts the steps are: wash, add to rapidly boiling water, simmer from 1 to 5 minutes, pour out the water, set aside to cool.

- For steaming broccoli, cauliflower, Brussels sprouts and similar vegetables the steps are: wash, cut if needed, steam, let cool. Steaming times are between 3 to 10 minutes depending on your preference. Steaming is done with a pot of boiling water and a steaming basket.

- If cooking times are relatively short, there is little difference in the result between these methods.

Care must be taken not to overcook these vegetables, as they will quickly become mushy. Cook just enough to remove the raw edge, but still leave them crisp. Alternatively cut Brussels sprouts and broccoli can be stir fried, pan fried or sauteed with other food.

Cooking beans

Most larger beans should be soaked from 4 to 10 hours before cooking and then rinsed. Soaking beans initiates a chemical change that breaks down some of the hard to digest complex carbohydrates. This causes the beans to be easier to digest and produce less gas in your digestive system. I have met people who do not eat beans, because they thought that beans were "incompatible with my digestive system and give me too much gas". With beans that are soaked before cooking, they were surprised to find that they had no such problems. Small legumes like lentils should be rinsed, but do not need to be soaked.

Sweeter beans, such as adzuki, black eyed peas and mung beans are easiest to digest. Cooking beans with bay leaves, cumin, epazote or kombu will help to make them more digestible. Adding sweeteners such as honey or brown sugar will increase digestive problems.

Cooking procedure for beans that require soaking - Rinse and remove bad looking beans (if any), soak, rinse, add water, boil, simmer, drain, rinse.

If you are cooking beans that should be soaked, but are in a hurry you can boil them for 30 minutes instead of soaking them (and then simmer until tender), but it is much better to soak them because of the chemical breakdown of complex carbs we talked about at the beginning of this section.

Cooking procedure for beans that do not require soaking - Rinse and remove bad looking beans (if any), add water, boil, simmer, drain, rinse.

The amount of water to add - In general, most beans will require 4 cups of water for one cup of beans (8 cups of water for a 1 pound bag of beans). Too much water will not hurt, because the beans will only absorb what they need and the rest will be poured out after cooking anyway.

Soaking and cooking times - Listed below are soaking and cooking guidelines for various types of dried beans. Each brand of beans are grown under different conditions, so the exact cook times will vary considerably. Try a few beans half way through the cooking time and every 10 minutes after that, to see if they are soft enough according to your preferences. If they are ready, rinse them and serve. Remember the exact cooking time for the next time you cook them.

- Adzuki beans   Soak=no, boil=10 min, simmer=1/2 to 1 hrs
- Baby lima beans   Soak=yes, boil=10 min, simmer=¾ to 1 hrs
- Butter beans   Soak=yes, boil=10 min, simmer=1 hrs
- Black beans   Soak=yes, boil=10 min, simmer=1 hrs
- Black eyed peas   Soak=no, boil=10 min, simmer=3/4 hrs
- Cannellini beans   Soak=no, boil=10 min, simmer=3/4 hrs
- Chickpeas   Soak=yes, boil=10 min, simmer=1/2 hrs
- Desi chickpeas   Soak=yes, boil=10 min, simmer=3/4 hrs
- Fava beans   Soak=yes, boil=10 min, simmer=1 hrs
- Mayocoba beans   Soak=yes, boil=10 min, simmer=1 hrs
- Mung beans   Soak=no, boil=10 min, simmer=1 hrs
- Navy beans   Soak=yes, boil=10 min, simmer=1 hrs
- Pinto beans   Soak=yes, boil=10 min, simmer=1.5 hrs
- Red beans   Soak=yes, boil=10 min, simmer=1.5 hrs
- Kidney beans   Soak=yes, boil=10 min, simmer=1 hrs
- Soybeans   Soak=no, boil=10 min, simmer=3 hrs

Phytohaemagglutinin - Some larger beans (in particular kidney beans and to a lesser extent fava beans) have a naturally occurring toxin (phytohaemagglutinin) that is destroyed by boiling. These beans must be boiled for at least 30 minutes before simmering, if they have not been soaked. If they have been soaked for 8 hours, they should be boiled for at least 10 minutes. Do not cook larger beans, such as kidney beans in a slow cooker without boiling them first on the stove. A slow cooker does not get hot enough to neutralize phytohaemagglutinin and the lower heat of a slow cooker will actually increase the amount of phytohaemagglutinin by up to five times. Phytohaemagglutinin poisoning will usually cause nausea and vomiting within a few hours, followed by diarrhea.

Cooking lentils and split peas

Lentils and split peas do not have to be soaked. Each brand of lentils and peas are slightly different, so the exact cook times will vary. Try some half way through the cooking time and every 5 minutes after that, to see if they are soft enough according to your preferences. If they are ready, rinse and serve. Remember the exact cooking time for the next time you cook them.

Cooking procedure for lentils and peas - Rinse, add water (1 cup lentils or peas to 4 cups or more of water), boil for 5 minutes, simmer for 25 to 45 minutes until tender, drain, rinse and serve.

Cooking rice

Cooking rice can done by three different methods, absorption, steaming or boiling. Although most instructions call for adding salt to rice, it has no effect on cooking and should be added after the meal is prepared and not during cooking.

Absorption is the most popular method used for cooking rice and the method used by most electric rice cookers. Some rice has surface starch that can be removed by rinsing. If you rinse, the rice grains will remain separate after cooking. If you do not rinse, the rice will stick together because of the starch. You can tell if there is starch by rinsing sample of the rice, if the water is milky looking there is starch.

Absorption cooking procedure for rice - Rinse, add water, cook, serve. A specific amount of water is measured for a set amount of rice, as shown in the table below. The water and rice are brought to a boil and the temperature is then reduced to a simmer. Cooking is complete when the water has been absorbed by the rice. The cook times shown below are approximate, so you must watch closely and turn off the stove when there is no more water or the rice on the bottom of the pot will burn. A rice cooker does this automatically.

- Basmati   1 cup rice to 2 cups water, soak 30 min, rinse, simmer 30 min
- Black   1 cup rice to 2 cups water, simmer 30 min
- Brown   1 cup rice to 2 cups water, simmer 30-40 min
- Jasmine   1 cup rice to 2 cups water, simmer 30 min
- Parboiled   1 cup rice to 2 cups water, simmer 30 min
- Texmati   1 cup rice to 2 cups water, simmer 20 min
- Wild   1 cup rice to 2 cups water, simmer 40 min

Steaming procedure for rice - Steaming works best for sticky types of rice. The rice is first soaked for one hour and drained before being steamed for 30 to 40 minutes. A steaming pot and steaming basket are used.

Boiling procedure for rice - Boiling produces results similar to absorption. Use 1 cup of rice to 4 cups of water. Rinsing before cooking is optional. The rice is added to boiling water and occasionally stirred. Cook until tender, this takes from 20 to 30 minutes for most types of rice. Pour out the remaining water before serving.

Cooking grains

Most grains such as millet, quinoa, pearl barley, bulgur wheat, wheat berries and kamut should be rinsed until the water runs clear. Add 1 cup of grain to 2-1/2 cups of water. Boil and reduce to a simmer. Cook time is 5 to 40 minutes, depending on the type of grain. Test occasionally and stop cooking when grains are chewy (not too hard and not too soft). Pour out excess water, no need to rinse before serving.

Cooking Cassava (yuca root)

Cassava (yuca root) must be peeled before cooking to remove the thick skin and any wax that has been applied to preserve them. This is best done with a vegetable peeler. Cassava must be properly prepared and cooked, raw cassava has cyanogenic glycosides that produce toxic cyanide. After peeling, slice it into small sections (like splitting a log) and simmer for 30 minutes. This will detoxify the sweet cassava that is available in most grocery stores. Bitter cassava produces 50 times more cyanide and should not be cooked at home.

Cooking root vegetables

Root vegetables such as carrots, beets, turnip, rutabaga, radish and parsnip can be boiled, pressure cooked, steamed, baked or stir fried. They can be cooked plain and seasoned later or cooked in a broth or stock. After washing, cut them into pieces so that they will cook evenly. Cooking time is generally 10 minutes or longer depending on the size of the pieces being cooked, they should be cooked to the point they are tender enough to eat.

Making soup

Soup is one of the easiest things to make. Soups can be clear or thick.

Thick - Thick soup starts with a thickening agent of some type, this can be flour, grains, lentils, split peas, rice, squashes, potatoes, sweet potatoes, tomatoes, etc. Making thick soup is a two part process. First cook the food to be used as the thickening agent and then put it in the blender to make a puree. Once it is blended, put it in a soup pot and add additional ingredients and seasonings of your choice. Simmer until the desired taste and consistency is obtained. Some popular ingredients are mixed vegetables, lima beans, green peas, cubed tomato, stewed tomato, potato cubes, tofu or tempeh cubes, etc.

Clear - Clear soup starts with a broth or stock of some type. This can be purchased or made. Several companies sell organic broths and stocks with healthy ingredients. Making clear soup is a two part process. First; prepare or make the stock. Making stock is covered in the next section. Second; once the stock is simmering add additional ingredients and seasonings as desired. Continue to simmer until the desired taste and consistency is obtained. Some popular ingredients are mixed vegetables, kale, spinach, lima beans, black eyed peas, cubed tomato, stewed tomato, potato cubes, tofu or tempeh cubes, etc.

Making stock and Broth

Stock and broth are made by boiling vegetables or meat. Stock and broth are similar, stock is usually strained and broth still has some small parts of the vegetables or meat remaining. The easiest way to make stock and broth is by saving the cooking water from your organic vegetables or meat (or both). Alternatively you can boil a small quantity of organic vegetables and save the water. For stock use a coarse strainer or grate, for broth use a fine strainer to remove all solids. Any kind of vegetables or meats can be used to make stock and broth.

Making stew

Making stew is the same as making thick soup, just use less water so that the puree is thicker. Most stews will have more solid food in them such as vegetable cubes, chunks of tempeh and tofu, etc.

Bread and baked goods

Not everyone has the time to bake bread and other baked foods, but if you try it you may find that it is easier than you thought. Baking is fun and you can bake healthier foods than you can buy, and put in your own custom ingredients.

How bread is made - Making bread and baked goods (such as muffins and rolls), starts with flour, water and a leavening agent that are mixed to make dough. The dough can be mixed by hand, but is easier with a powered mixer. One pound of flour will make about one loaf of bread. After mixing, the dough is baked at 350 to 425 F. Without leavening, the bread will be hard and flat, like flat bread or matzah. Leavening causes gas bubbles to form in the dough and this makes the dough rise (expand). For home baking, yeast or baking powder are usually used as the leavening agent. There are many ingredients that can be added to the dough, such as salt, nuts, seeds, berries, fruit, concentrated fruit juice, whole grains, nut butter, malt extract, molasses, etc. The kind of flour and ingredients that are used determines the type of bread or baked good that is made.

Breads are processed - All breads are a processed food to some degree, ranging from lightly processed in the case of old-world breads made with stone ground whole grain flour, to American white bread which is heavily processed. When you make bread you have control of the ingredients and can make the healthiest bread from high quality ingredients. However, keep in mind that lightly processed baked goods still have a higher energy density than the whole foods that were used to make the ingredients. For this reason baked goods should only be eaten occasionally, unless you require a higher energy food, for example for hiking or cycling long distances or other prolonged strenuous physical activity.

Making healthy baked goods - Baking healthy breads without oil, fat and sugar, will take some effort. The section "Flour" in chapter five explains about stone ground whole grain flour. There are some companies that specialize in stone ground whole grain flours and other healthy ingredients, a few of these are listed in the section "Fresh, frozen, dried or canned?" in chapter six. There is no way to make healthy breads and baked goods that look and taste like the processed varieties common to the American diet, don't waste your time trying. It is better to start with healthy recipes, rather than trying to adapt existing recipes. Baked goods made from whole grains and healthy ingredients will be a different type of food with it's own appeal and qualities.

More on baking bread - If you are interested in healthy baking a great book on the subject is Healthy Bread in Five Minutes a Day: 100 New Recipes Featuring Whole Grains, Fruits, Vegetables, and Gluten-Free Ingredients, by Zoe Francois & Jeff Hertzberg M.D.

Sprouts and sprouting

When a dry seed receives water and starts to grow, it produces a seedling. This is known as germination or sprouting. Sprouting normally takes about one to four days. Sprouting is a handy way to create fresh food from dry food. Dry seeds can be stored for long periods of time and sprouted when fresh food is needed, such as during the winter months. Sprouting is easy to do and can be done using a sprouting jar right in your kitchen.

There are nutritional and economic advantages to sprouting. Sprouting causes a substantial increase in nutrients, including many vitamins. The process of sprouting consumes starches and fiber and causes the sprouts have a higher percentage of protein. Cost wise there is an increase in the food value of the sprouted seeds. Sprouting is a good way to stretch your food budget.

What to sprout - Any type of viable seed, bean or nut can be sprouted. Some popular examples are:

- Legumes - Chickpea, Mung bean, Soybean, Alfalfa, Lentil, Pea, etc.
- Grains - Brown rice, Barley, Oat, Wheat, Corn, Quinoa, Amaranth, Buckwheat, etc.

- Seeds & nuts - Flaxseed, Hazelnut, Linseed, Peanut, sesame, sunflower, almond, etc.

What not to sprout - Some seeds are not suitable for sprouting, because they are poisonous. Some examples of poisonous seeds are eggplant, rhubarb, tomato, potato and paprika. Some seeds are meant for planting only and have been treated with pesticides and poisonous chemical coatings to prevent animals and insects from eating them. Never sprout seeds that are sold specifically for planting.

Bacteria issues - Bacteria such as salmonella growing during the sprouting process, can be a concern. Bacteria can originate from the soil or fertilizer where the seeds were originally grown. Cooking the sprouts before eating is one way to kill bacteria. It is a good idea to check the internet or buy a book about sprouting to learn sprouting methods that avoid the growth of bacteria.

Sprouting procedure example - There are several techniques for sprouting, depending on the type of seed, this example is for soybeans and is done in a sprouting jar with a perforated lid.

1. Fill the jar 3/4th full with beans.
2. Rinse several times with water.
3. Fill the jar with water and soak for 8 hours.
4. Rinse and leave the jar upside down to drain.
5. Rinse and drain twice a day.
6. After the beans are sprouted wash thoroughly.

Fermentation

Fermentation uses microorganisms such as yeast and bacteria, to convert the carbohydrates in food into alcohol, carbon dioxide and organic acid. This changes the taste and consistency of the food. Some examples of foods that are made using fermentation are bread, beer, pickles, sauerkraut, kimchee, soy sauce, wine and vinegar. Natural fermentation occurs in many fruits and vegetables. For example, grapes and blueberries usually have a white or tan powdery looking substance covering them. This is naturally occurring yeast.

Many types of fermented foods can be made at home. To learn more about fermentation and how to make fermented foods, a good book on the subject is "Wild Fermentation: The Flavor, Nutrition, and Craft of Live-Culture Foods Reclaiming Domesticity from a Consumer Culture" by Sandor Ellix Katz.

Substitutions and measurements

Teaspoons & Tablespoons - As a unit of measurement for dry ingredients, teaspoons and tablespoons can cause problems, especially for critical ingredients such as baking powder, baking soda or yeast. There are three possible measurements, level, rounded and heaping. A level spoon is flat to the top of the spoon. Heaping is the maximum amount possible heaped on the spoon. Rounded is in between. When a recipe does not specifically state the type of spoon, use a rounded spoon.

Substitutions in recipes - If you are converting a baking recipe from processed ingredients to healthy ingredients, the following substitutions may help:

- To substitute for fat, butter or oil; use applesauce, sweet potatoes, white beans, pumpkin, pear sauce, mashed banana, avocado or nut butter. Canned foods are a handy source for these ingredients because they are already cooked and ready to use.

- To substitute for sugar or artificial sweetener; use turbinado sugar, maple syrup, honey, frozen orange juice or frozen grape juice.

- To substitute for milk; use almond milk, soy milk or rice milk.

- To substitute for one egg; use one tablespoon ground flaxseed mixed with two tablespoons of water.

Frequently Asked Questions

Question: I have heard that cooking and baking at high temperatures can cause the formation of acrylamide and other carcinogenic substances.

Answer: Yes. The temperatures must be high enough to cause browning or burning for acrylamide to form and it depends on the composition of the food being cooked. Foods that are high in starches such as potatoes or wheat flour, cause the formation of acrylamides more than some other foods. Some examples of foods that are cooked at high temperatures and are high in acrylamide are processed foods, fast food, fried foods including french fries, bread crust, toasted bread, molasses, soy sauce, coffee, etc. In general the more brown or black the outside of the food becomes, the more acrylamide that is formed. In the case of blackened food or food that has been burned or charred, other carcinogenic chemicals and substances besides acrylamide are also formed.

This creates a problem in cooking, because smoking, toasting, baking, barbecuing or otherwise cooking food at high temperatures produces great tasting food that is used in many cuisines. Unfortunately there is no easy fix for this problem, you have to make a choice between the eating food that is cooked in this way or protecting yourself from these harmful substances and chemicals. Personally I have limited my intake of foods that contain acrylamide and eliminated the worst offending foods from my diet completely. To learn more about acrylamide, Wikipedia is a good place to start, with links to many sources.

8 - Breakfast

This chapter covers breakfast dishes, see the section "Balanced breakfast" at the end of the chapter for ideas to combine breakfast dishes into meals.

It's good to base breakfast on foods that provide long term energy like oatmeal or other types of hot cereal. This will give you the energy you need for most of the day and keep you from getting hungry before lunch. That being said, our first topic is, hot cereal!

Hot cereal

There are many types of hot cereals, most are made from grains, oatmeal is the most popular. Hot cereals are best when eaten with fruit, nuts, seeds and other toppings. A bowl of hot cereal topped with fruit and nuts, is a complete breakfast that can be made in a few minutes.

Adding 2 or 3 tablespoons of flaxseed and a tablespoon of nutritional yeast to your bowl of hot cereal will take care of most of your daily omega 3 fatty acid and vitamin B12 requirements. Not everyone likes the taste and consistency of flaxseed and nutritional yeast in their hot cereal, but if you do, this works out well.

Oatmeal - Old fashioned rolled oats or quick cooking rolled oats should be used. The difference is that the quick cooking oats are cut into pieces and rolled thinner, this enables them to absorb water faster and decreases the cooking time. Avoid the instant oatmeal, most instant oatmeal is processed and has unwanted ingredients. Oatmeal, like any hot cereal can be cooked on the stove or in the microwave oven. There are many things that can be added to oatmeal, experiment to find what you like.

Other hot cereals - Grains such as Buckwheat groats, Barley, Bulgur wheat, Wheat berries, Grits (polenta), 10 grain, Soy grits, Farina (Cream of Wheat), Amaranth, and other hot cereals make a good alternative to oatmeal. Try mixing two grains to add variety. One of my favorite sources for hot cereals is Bob's Red Mill. Their cereals are sold in most stores and online.

Microwave cooking - To cook a single bowl of hot cereal start with ½ cup cereal with 1 cup water. Adjust the amount of water to achieve the consistency that you like. Add flaxseed if you like, cook for 1-½ to 2-½ minutes (depending on how powerful your microwave is). Let it stand for another minute or two before adding fruit and toppings.

Stove top cooking - For two people start with 2 cups of water, bring it to a boil. Add 1 cup cereal. Cook for 2 to 5 minutes, until it has the desired consistency. Experiment with the cooking time and the amount water, until you perfect your hot cereal. Try adding ingredients (like nuts) before cooking or after cooking, to see how you like it best. Let it stand a few minutes before adding fruit and toppings.

Toppings and ingredients for hot cereal - Use any combination of these toppings and ingredients to jazz up your hot cereal:

- Frozen or fresh fruit; Banana, Mango, Pineapple, Blueberries, Blackberries, Apple, Grapefruit, Peach, Pear, Strawberries, Grapes, cherries, Frozen mixed berries, Raisins, Figs, Dates, Kiwi, Dried fruit of all types, etc.
- Nuts & seeds; Walnuts, Almonds, Sunflower seeds, Pecans, Chia seed, Flaxseed, etc.
- Other toppings; Molasses, Ceylon cinnamon, Nutmeg, Nutritional yeast, Frozen orange or grape juice, Sea salt, Honey, Soy milk, Almond milk, granola, etc.

Cold cereal

Granola - Most commercially available granola has sweeteners and other unwanted ingredients such as oil, cane juice, sugar, high fructose corn syrup, etc. In other words, store bought granola is just another processed food. Even the granola that is sold in the bulk bins at health food stores has too much oil and cane juice (a sweetener). For this reason it is best to make your own granola. Fortunately it is easy to make granola, just put your ingredients on an oven tray and bake for 15 to 45 minutes at 300 F. You will end up saving money and making better granola than any store bought type. You will have to play around with the temperature and baking times for your exact mix of ingredients.

- Zoie's chewy granola - This recipe makes about 10 cups of granola. 6 cups oats, 1/4th cup Ceylon cinnamon, 1/4th cup nutmeg, 2 cups sunflower seeds, 8 oz honey + 1 cup water (mixed), 8 oz chopped walnuts. Mix all ingredients and spread the mix on oven trays. Bake for 30 to 45 minutes at 300 F. After baking, add 2 cups of raisins. Alternatively you can reduce the amount of walnuts and add almonds, cashews, pecans or other types of nuts.

Cold hot-cereal! - That's right, you can use any type of hot cereal as a cold cereal. Instead of cooking it, soak the hot cereal overnight (or at least for several hours, depending on the type of grain). Just add water the night before and by the time you get up in the morning your cereal is ready to eat. This works great for camping or traveling when you don't have a stove or don't feel like messing around with cooking. This technique is also great for road trips or at work, just use a sealed container instead of a bowl.

- Cold-hot Oatmeal - This makes enough for one serving. ½ cup rolled oats, 3 tablespoons ground flaxseed or chia seed, 1-¼ cup almond milk, 1 teaspoon Ceylon cinnamon. Mix and cover your bowl, put it in the refrigerator overnight. In the morning top with banana slices or other fruit.

- Buckwheat cereal - Soak 1 cups of buckwheat groats in 1 cup of vanilla almond milk or vanilla soy milk overnight. In the morning add fruit, cinnamon, chia seeds, nutmeg or nuts as you like.

Smoothies

A smoothie is a thick beverage made in a blender. Almost any type of food can be used to make a smoothie, including fruit, vegetables, ice, peanut butter, honey, soy milk, green tea, etc. Smoothies are different from juice and juicing, because smoothies are made in a blender and the blades of the blender chop the ingredients, no part of the ingredients are filtered or removed. This leaves all of the fiber and pulp in the smoothie, which is good. No refinement takes place and the energy profile of the ingredients is unchanged.

Making a smoothie is simple, just put the ingredients in the blender and turn it on. Let it run until the right thickness and consistency is achieved. If it is too thick, add a little water. Making smoothies takes some playing around before you find the ingredients that you like and the right amount of liquid to add.

People who want more raw vegetables in their diet, but don't like eating them can put their raw vegetables in smoothies. In this way a substantial amount of raw vegetables can be consumed without it being very noticeable. As long as the smoothie is consumed immediately or kept at a low temperature until it is consumed, there is little or no nutritional penalty, in fact the blending action makes some nutrients more bio available.

Smoothies are a good replacement for snack food, because they are quick to make and do not require cooking. They are easy to take with you if you have a bottle or thermos. Some of my favorite ingredients are bananas, strawberries, kale, crushed ice, broccoli, hummus and peanut butter.

The following are some ideas for various types of smoothies:

Strawberry smoothie - Serves 2 people. 2 cups chopped strawberries, ½ cup cooked oatmeal, 1 cup vanilla soy milk, 4 ice cubes, ¼ cup frozen orange juice.

Kale smoothie - Serves 2 people. 3 cups chopped kale, 1 cup broccoli, ½ cup chopped walnuts, 1 tablespoon molasses, 4 ice cubes, 4 cups vanilla soy milk.

Kale & pineapple smoothie - Serves 2 people. 3 cups chopped kale, 1 cup pineapple, ½ cup chopped walnuts, 1 tablespoon molasses, 4 ice cubes, 4 cups vanilla soy milk.

Banana smoothie - Serves 2 people. 3 bananas, ½ cup cooked oatmeal or other hot cereal, 1-½ cup vanilla soy milk, 4 ice cubes, ¼ cup frozen orange juice.

Broccoli & banana smoothie - Serves 2 people. 2 bananas, 2 cups broccoli, ½ cup cooked oatmeal or other hot cereal, 1-½ cup vanilla soy milk, 4 ice cubes, ¼ cup frozen orange juice.

Pumpkin & spinach smoothie - Serves 2 people. 1 banana, ½ cup canned pumpkin, 2 cups spinach, 1 cup vanilla soy milk or vanilla almond milk, ¼ cup frozen orange juice, one tablespoon molasses, 4 ice cubes, 1 teaspoon Ceylon cinnamon.

Simple breakfast dishes

Applesauce - There are several brands of home style applesauce on the market that do not have sweeteners added, the only ingredient is apples. Applesauce with Ceylon cinnamon is one of my favorites.

Baked hash browns - Use a spiralizer or food processor to make potato strands, bake or fry with just a touch of oil.

Black bean patties - There are some healthy organic black bean patties on the market, or you can make your own (see recipe in chapter nine). Fried black bean patties go great with pancakes or can be used to make breakfast sandwiches.

Breakfast vegetable soup - In many cuisines, breakfast soups are a daily menu item, especially in cold weather. See chapter seven for preparation and cooking of soup.

Breakfast vegetable stew - You can combine soup with beans or lentils and tomato to make a breakfast stew. This is great on cold winter days.

Fruits, berries & nut bowls - Mixed fruit bowls with sliced or cubed fruits, berries and nuts are great for breakfast. One of my favorites is pineapple, grapes and walnuts.

Fruit sauces - Fruit sauces such as pear sauce and cranberry sauce make a great addition to breakfast. If you are buying them canned make sure that they do not have added sugar or high fructose corn syrup.

Onions, bell peppers and mushrooms - Fried or sauteed, onions, bell peppers and mushrooms make a good breakfast combination. Together with a fried black bean patty and some fruit and you have a full breakfast.

Onions, spinach and mushrooms - Fried or sauteed, onions, spinach and mushrooms will put some green leafy vegetables in your breakfast in a way that still seems like breakfast! Add some tofu or a fried black bean patty and some fruit and you have a full breakfast.

Plantains - Plantains can be boiled, baked or fried. Plantains and tofu fried with honey or molasses are great breakfast dish.

Nut butter and sliced fruit sandwiches - Any kind of nut butter can be used, such as peanut butter or almond butter. You can even use hummus. The fruit can be bananas, pineapple, apple, mango, nectarine, pitted cherries, raisins, dates, dried fruit, etc.

Stir fried tofu or tempeh - A great side dish to go with pancakes. Fried tofu or tempeh go good with salsa and avocado.

Sliced tomato and tofu - This can be a hot or cold dish. Works well with some flavored vinegar or vinegar and ground peppercorn.

Sweet potato cakes - Microwave medium sized sweet potatoes and slice them into rounds (like cutting a log). Pan fry the rounds with seasoning such as Molasses, Ceylon cinnamon, Frozen orange juice, etc.

Recipes

The following recipes use the least processed ingredients possible, but could take some adjustment to meet your expectations. It may take several attempts, depending on the type of flour and other ingredients you use. See the section on baking in chapter seven for ideas troubleshooting baked goods.

Blueberry pancakes - This recipe makes 8 large blueberry pancakes. 1 cup of blueberries are used, they are added in step four so that they do not get crushed in the blender. You can use strawberries instead if you want strawberry pancakes.

Mix the following dry ingredients together in a large bowl:

- 1-½ cups whole grain flour of your choice.
- ¼ cup ground flaxseed.
- 2 teaspoons baking powder.
- ½ teaspoon baking soda.
- ¼ teaspoon salt.

Blend the following wet ingredients in a blender:

- ½ cup water.
- 2 mashed bananas.
- 1 cups applesauce.
- ¼ cup frozen grape juice.
- 2 tablespoons molasses.

Mix the wet and dry ingredients using a mixing bowl or power mixer: Add the wet ingredients first and then slowly add the dry ingredients while mixing to make your batter.

After the batter is mixed, gently stir in one cup of blueberries before the batter is poured into the muffin tray.

Use cooking spray or a little oil to lightly oil the pan or griddle. Use medium-high heat.

Chia seed squares - This recipe makes 24 squares.

Mix the following ingredients together using a mixing bowl or power mixer:

- 1-½ cups whole grain flour of your choice.

- 1 cup chia seeds.

- 3 teaspoons baking powder.

- ½ teaspoon salt.

- 1 teaspoon Ceylon cinnamon.

- 1-½ cup vanilla soy milk or vanilla almond milk.

Bake: Use cooking spray or a little oil to lightly coat the baking pan before filling about 1 inch with batter. Bake for about 25 minutes at 325 F and check to see if done.

Drinks

Tea - Try Earl Gray or English Breakfast tea in the morning. Hot tea is very healthy. Green tea is the best and has the least caffeine. Black tea is a good replacement for coffee, it is better health wise and has much less caffeine than coffee. Tea should never get boring, there are many kinds of herbal tea and flavored tea.

- Bush tea - Rooibos tea has immune system building properties as do turmeric and ginger. This tea is great anytime, but really helps when you are not feeling so good. Load a tea infuser with loose rooibos tea leaves, finely sliced turmeric root and finely sliced ginger root. You can buy the turmeric root and ginger root in the produce section of most grocery stores and use a slicer peel off the skin. Use a julienne slicer to finely slice the root. Lower the tea infuser into a pot of boiling water until the tea is the desired strength. Add some squeezed lemon.

- Citrus tea - Start with almost any tea such as black tea or green tea, add fresh squeezed orange, grapefruit, or lemon to taste.

Juice - Store bought juice is a processed food and should be avoided. In the multi-stage process of making juice most of the beneficial fiber and other important parts of the fruit are filtered and removed which increases the energy density and destroys much of the nutritional value. As far as home made juice, most home juicers also filter or remove the pulp removing much of the nutritional value. Unfiltered fresh squeezed juice is OK, but why not just eat the whole fruit or add it to a smoothie instead?

Switchel - A great sports drink or drink to cool you down in hot weather is switchel. It is made from water, vinegar and ginger. Some people add lemon juice, salt or molasses.

Snack bars & trail mix

In a number of circumstances you may find yourself in a hurry and need to grab something quick from home or the grocery store to give yourself some energy. An alternative instead of getting something completely unhealthy, is snack bars or trail mix. It is best to combine them with fruit such as bananas, oranges, pears or apples.

Snack bars - Snack bars or breakfast bars can be made in your kitchen or purchased. Watch the list of ingredients if you are buying snack bars, most snack bars are nutritionally bad, almost as bad as candy. There are a few brands that are making an effort to be healthy and use less processed ingredients such as Clif Bar, Luna and Odwalla.

Raisin breakfast bars - Breakfast bars and power bars are easy to make. This recipe makes about 16 bars. 1 cup raisins, 1-¼ cup of one minute quick oats, ¼ cup ground flaxseed, 1 cup chopped walnuts, ½ cup pitted dates, 1 cup dried mango or apricot, ½ cup frozen orange juice, ½ cup whole grain flour. Use a power mixer to mix the ingredients. Add water if needed until the consistency is like thick dough. Cook in a medium bread pan for 30 minutes at 300 F. After cooling use a bread knife to cut into bars.

Trail mix - You can buy or make your own trail mix. If you are buying trail mix, watch the ingredients closely, trail mix varies from being junk food to being totally healthy. In general, trail mix that is sold in the bulk bins at stores like Whole Foods Markets is better quality and lower priced than the trail mix that comes in plastic packaging and is sold by name brand suppliers in the regular grocery store. Making your own trail mix is easy, just combine the ingredients, toasting is optional.

Balanced breakfast

A balanced diet consists of vegetables + fruits & berries + legumes + seeds & nuts + grains & starches. Your breakfast does not have to be balanced if food that is not included in breakfast is made up for later in the day. Specifically, some people do not like eating green vegetables during breakfast. Alternatively, a good way to get your green vegetables during breakfast is to put them in a smoothie.

Most people like to have a light and quick breakfast such as a bowl of cereal with some fruit on top. In this case you can eat some additional greens later in the day and still maintain a balanced diet.

The following are some ideas for breakfast meals:

- Hot cereal with fruit and nuts + Pineapple & kale smoothie.
- Chia seed muffins + Fruit & nut bowl + Broccoli & banana smoothie.
- Plantains + Fried Onions, bell peppers and mushrooms + Oatmeal smoothie.
- Plantains + Fried Onions, spinach and mushrooms + Oatmeal smoothie.
- Breakfast vegetable stew + Berries & nut bowl.
- Blueberry pancakes + Black bean patty - Pumpkin & spinach smoothie.

9 - Lunch & Dinner

Instead of a traditional and complicated main course, most meals in this book are made from two or more simple side dishes. This allows day to day cooking to be done quickly without recipes. Ideas for combining these side dishes to form balanced meals are covered in the section "Balanced lunch & dinner" at the end of the chapter.

These dishes are basic and are meant as a starting place to be built on. As you develop your own style, you will discover more sophisticated ways of preparing, combining and serving whole foods. Don't be afraid to experiment. When you are ready to get more advanced, or if you need some ideas for recipes there is a list of books in chapter twelve that will help.

Whole foods keep well in sealed containers when refrigerated. Instead of preparing food for a single meal, it makes sense to prepare food for several meals at a time, or even enough for several days. This will cut down on the time spent cooking and provide healthy foods to snack on any time you are hungry. You can also take this food with you for lunch.

Lunch & dinner side dishes

The following list of side dishes illustrates the point that a whole food diet does not need to be boring! Two or more side dishes can be combined to make a complete meal, and some of them (like stir fried vegetables) can be a complete meal by themselves. Many of these dishes have similar preparation methods and cooking times, so it is easy to make several of them at the same time.

Appetizers - Sliced fruit, fruit bowls or fruit salads make a great appetizer and an easy way to include a portion of fruit in the lunch and dinner meal.

Asparagus - Asparagus is best boiled or steamed. If boiled, you can use the following method to keep the tender tops from being overcooked. Asparagus normally comes in a bunch with rubber bands holding it together. Take the rubber band off of the bottom but leave the top bound. Boil a pot of water and then set the asparagus standing up in the water with the bottoms under the water. Let the bottoms cook for about 5 minutes and then take the rubber band off the top and allow the asparagus to entirely submerge in the boiling water. Let it boil another few minutes until the tops are tender.

Baked vegetables - Almost any combination of vegetables can be baked in a baking pan. Sliced squash, onion, tomatoes, eggplant and green or red pepper makes a good combination. Just wash, slice and bake for 20 or 30 minutes at 300 F. Use more cook time if needed. You can use seasonings and sauces before or after baking.

Beans - Dried beans must be cooked or sprouted (or both), this is covered in chapter seven. Canned beans are pre-cooked and can be eaten cold or heated. Beans with added sweeteners such as honey or brown sugar are much harder to digest and cause gas. Beans can be seasoned in various ways. We like them with chili pepper, bay leaf, tomato sauce, chopped yellow onions, and dash of sea salt. There are many other ways to season beans, you should experiment until you find the seasonings that suit your taste.

Bean salads - There are many variations of cold bean salads, some favorites are as follows:

- Hot Lima; lima beans, desi chick peas, red wine vinegar and hot pepper.
- Traditional; Kidney beans, cut green beans and flavored vinaigrette.
- Texas Caviar; black eyed peas pickled in vinaigrette.
- Chickpea; chickpeas, onion, ground peppercorn and flavored vinaigrette.
- Three bean salad; white beans, black eyed peas, kidney beans, flavored vinaigrette.
- Hot Black; black beans, desi chickpeas, red wine vinegar and chopped jalapeno pepper.

Broccoli, cauliflower and Brussels sprouts (individually or together) - Broccoli, cauliflower and Brussels sprouts are best boiled or steamed and seasoned after cooking or served unseasoned. Once on your dinner plate you can use black pepper, sauces, soy sauce or mixed seasonings such as Mrs Dash. How to boil and steam broccoli, cauliflower and Brussels sprouts is covered in chapter seven. Alternatively, sliced Brussels sprouts and broccoli can also be stir fried, pan fried or sauteed with other food.

Canned foods - Canned pumpkin, tomato paste, tomato sauce, mixed beans, green peas, beets, cranberry sauce, and black beans are some of my favorite side dishes when I am in a hurry. Canned side dishes come in handy if you have some food that was prepared previously in containers but are missing a side dish to round out the meal. In this case, you can just open the can instead of cooking. Canned green vegetables are generally over cooked and over salted, fresh or frozen green vegetables are preferred. Always check the list of ingredients of canned food to make sure there are no unwanted preservatives or chemicals used, if there are, try another brand.

Canned mixed greens, yams and sweet potatoes tend to have sweeteners, heavy amounts of salt and artificial ingredients. Some canned foods like boiled peanuts, some beans and yams can be simply drained and rinsed to remove most of the salt.

Canned soup, chili, chunky soup or other heavily flavored canned food can be used as a topping or flavoring ingredient for other foods. I was once in a hurry preparing dinner for guests and added a can of creamy split pea soup to a pot of lentils for flavoring and got more compliments than any food I had cooked in months!

Cassava (yuca root) - Cassava makes a great alternative to potatoes. Boiled and mashed cassava tastes like mashed potatoes with some kind of buttery dressing, but cassava doesn't need any dressing, that's just how it tastes. How to cook cassava is covered in chapter seven.

Coleslaw - Coleslaw is a side dish made from cabbage, that is cut into strands with a spiralizer or food processor and dressed with a vinaigrette dressing. It can be allowed to pickle for a few days.

Corn - There are many types of organic corn that are more nutritious and have a real taste. The commercial monocrop corn that is sold in most grocery stores has most of the taste bred out of it. Corn on the cob can be boiled, steamed or baked in tin foil. Kernel corn can also be stir fried.

Couscous - Couscous is made from granules of durum wheat tan/white in color. It is fluffy and has a slight nutty flavor and texture. Couscous makes a great side dish by itself or can be added to other food. It is sold in dried form, in bags or in the bulk food section. To cook dried couscous put it in a bowl and pour in boiling water. Use 1 cup of couscous for 1-½ cups of water. Let it sit for 5 to 10 minutes and it will be ready to serve or you can add it to stir fried dishes.

Dried fruit and vegetables - You can buy or make dried (dehydrated) fruit and vegetables. There is usually an assortment in the bulk food section of stores such as Whole Foods Markets. Dried fruit and vegetables make a great ingredient or topping for salads and hot cereals. They are also good for trail mix. You can make your own dried fruit and vegetables by several methods including; oven, food dehydrator or sun exposure. See chapter twelve for recommended books about dehydrating food. Dried banana chips are a popular first dehydration project.

Fennel bulb - The bulb of the fennel plant looks kind of like an onion, but with a strong nutty flavor. You can cook it any of the ways that an onion can be cooked such as boiling, baking, frying. It makes a great side dish when grilled or stir fried. People may think it is onion and will wonder how you are able to get that kind of flavor out of an onion!

Fruits & berries - You can eat fruit individually as a side dish or you can make mixed fruit bowls with sliced or cubed fruits and berries. Another great idea is fruit and nut bowls such as pineapple, banana and walnuts.

Fruit sauces - Fruit sauces such as applesauce, pear sauce and cranberry sauce make a great side dish. Applesauce with Ceylon cinnamon is one of my favorites. If you are buying them from the store, make sure that they do not have added sugar or high fructose corn syrup.

Grains - Millet, quinoa, pearl barley, bulgur wheat, wheat berries, couscous and kamut are a great alternative to add variety to meals when rice gets boring. They can also be mixed with rice as a combination. Cooking grains is covered in chapter seven.

Green beans, green peas, snow peas, snap peas - These can be steamed, fried or boiled. They go great in stir fried mixed vegetables or with tofu or tempeh.

Greens and cabbage (individually or together) - Greens and cabbage are best boiled, this includes collard greens, kale, mustard greens, turnip greens, watercress, spinach, cabbage, purslane and amaranth. How to cook greens is covered in chapter seven. Chopped onion, chopped garlic or chopped fennel bulb can be added to greens during cooking for more flavor. Greens are usually seasoned at the end of cooking after some or all of the boiling water has been poured out. Some people prefer to serve greens without seasoning, so that they can be individually seasoned on the dinner plate. Greens can be seasoned various ways, such as with apple vinegar, ground black pepper, chopped yellow onions and a pinch of salt.

Guacamole - Mashed avocados are the main ingredient in guacamole. Other commonly used ingredients include tomato, cilantro, onion, lemon juice, garlic, chili pepper, etc. Guacamole is great on salads, in burritos and as a side dish that complements many types of foods. Guacamole is easy to make, just mash up some avocados and add other ingredients until it tastes the way you like it!

Hummus - Hummus makes a great side dish. You can buy some brands of healthy hummus, but it is better to make your own. See the recipe for hummus in the recipe section later in this chapter. There are many flavors of hummus, so it never has to get boring. Hummus has all of the good qualities of nut butters, but with less energy and fat content so you can eat far more hummus then nut butters without messing up your nutritional balance (take it from a recovering peanut butter and almond butter addict!).

Kimchi - Regular kimchi is made from napa cabbage that is cut into pieces and fermented with red chili pepper flakes. There other varieties of kimchi made with different vegetables. Kimchi is a Korean food and is available in most grocery stores (in jars), or you can make your own. Kimchi is made by lacto-fermentation (pickling) and has a long shelf life. Kimchi is high in salt, but if you plan for this you can use it as one of your sources of salt.

Lentils and split peas - Dried lentils and split peas must be cooked, this is covered in chapter seven. Lentils can be seasoned various ways, we like them with garlic, bay leaf, cumin and chopped yellow onions. Curry is also a popular seasoning for lentils. Some types of lentils, particularly the dark green or brown ones have a very nice flavor and may be better without any seasoning. Split peas generally don't need seasoning except possibly some ground pepper.

Meat - In this case we are including any of the following collectively as meat; Fish, Eggs, Seafood, Pork, Chicken, Beef, Bison, etc. Meat can be used as a side dish or as a garnishment, as is often done in Asian style cooking. I think that the best use of meat is as a flavoring and texture ingredient in other dishes such as stew, soup, greens, rice and beans, chicken fried rice, etc. When used as a flavoring and texture ingredient you get a lot of value from a small amount of meat, and that's a winning proposition from a nutritional standpoint.

Onions, bell peppers and mushrooms (individually or together) - These can be parboiled, stir fried or sauteed. Onions, bell peppers and mushrooms can be added to many dishes including soups, baked dishes and vegetable casseroles. Sauteed mushrooms can be seasoned with cooking wine, Worchester sauce and spices.

Onions, spinach and mushrooms - Fried or sauteed, onions, spinach and mushrooms are a great combination! Use some red wine or red wine vinegar when sauteing.

Plantains - Plantains can be boiled, baked or fried. Plain boiled plantains are great as a side dish. For baking and frying you can use almost any type of sauce or spices. Apple sauce and molasses fried plantains are an example.

Potatoes, Yams, etc - Tubers such as yams, potato, sweet potato and taro can be baked or boiled depending on your preference. Baking potatoes wrapped in aluminum foil will preserve some of the moisture. Wash thoroughly before cooking, because tubers usually receive a lot of pesticides, or better yet use organic tubers. Boiling may remove some of the pesticides. For individual meals, they can also be cooked in a microwave oven, this is much faster than baking or boiling. If you are microwaving whole tubers, make many small holes through the skin before cooking with a fork or knife to allow hot air to escape during cooking, otherwise they don't cook evenly and make strange whistling noises during cooking.

Rice - Cooking rice is covered in chapter seven. After being cooked, rice can be stir fried with other ingredients (such as vegetable fried rice) or added to a combination such as rice and beans or rice and lentils. Other ingredients can be mixed with rice after it is cooked to make Spanish rice, cilantro rice, etc.

Root vegetables - Root vegetables such as carrots, beets, turnip, rutabaga, radish and parsnip can be boiled, pressure cooked, steamed or baked. Root vegetables are great as a side dish or for use in soups and stews.

Salad - Forget traditional American style salads (iceberg lettuce, tomatoes, croutons, cheese, chicken or bacon drenched in processed salad dressing). Low fat "healthy" processed dressings don't help, instead of oil they use other processed ingredients. Avoiding processed dressings may be difficult at first, but you can make your own dressings. This is covered in the section "Dressings sauces and seasonings" later in this chapter. To take the place of croutons, cheese, bacon bits and other unhealthy ingredients use shiitake or portobello mushroom slices, chickpeas, nuts, sunflower seeds, etc.

When making a salad, start with greens such as kale, spinach, cabbage, romaine lettuce or mixed greens. After you have a bed of greens, add any combination of ingredients that you like, such as carrots, onion, cucumber, green peppers, tomatoes, grapes, raisins, cranberries, pineapple, other cubed fruit, chopped brussel sprouts, broccoli, mushrooms, snap peas, chickpeas, nuts, seeds, chick peas, desi chick peas, beans etc.

There are no rules in salad, no recipes are needed, experiment and have fun! If you don't like eating large pieces of vegetables, you can slice them into strands or strips similar to the way cabbage is cut for coleslaw. To do this quickly, you can use a food processor or a spiralizer (see chapter seven in the section "Optional cookware & equipment").

Sauerkraut - Sauerkraut is cabbage that is cut into strands and fermented. It is a German food and makes a great side dish. It is available in jars or you can make your own. Sauerkraut is made by lacto-fermentation, which is a form of pickling that is similar to the type of fermentation used to make kimchi and pickled cucumbers. Sauerkraut has a long shelf life. See chapter twelve for recommended books on fermentation. Sauerkraut is high in salt, but if you plan for this you can use it as one of your sources of salt.

Sprouted foods - Bean sprouts such as soy bean sprouts, Mung bean sprouts and lentil sprouts, make a great side dish raw or cooked. They can also be used as an ingredient for stir fried vegetables.

Squashes - Squashes such as zucchini, yellow squash, eggplant, acorn squash and pumpkin are best baked, stir fried or sauteed. After washing, cut into pieces and cook. Some squashes and pumpkin will need the seeds removed. Some types of squashes can be stuffed with rice and other ingredients before baking to make stuffed squash.

Stir fried vegetables - Get out the wok! Frozen and pre-washed stir fried vegetables are ready to be cooked, and are inexpensive and save time. Stir frying can be done in a fry pan or a wok, for one or two people, there is not much advantage to a wok over a small fry pan. Add some mushrooms, onions, hard tofu cubes or other ingredients for more variety. Instead of oil, or to reduce oil when stir frying, use vegetable broth or stock.

Stuffed, baked peppers - Bell peppers and other types of peppers, such as chili peppers can be stuffed with rice, chopped onion, cubed potato or sweet potato, etc. Other grains such as pearl barley, can be used with or instead of rice. After the pepper is stuffed, it is baked.

Tempeh - Tempeh can be eaten cold or cooked. It has more fiber and is less processed than tofu, it also has a stronger flavor than tofu (slightly nutty). Tempeh can be fried, sauteed or baked and can be made into patties and burgers. Tempeh burgers are a good alternative to black bean burgers.

Tofu - Tofu can be eaten cold or cooked. It can be cut into cubes and served plain or with soy sauce or other flavorings. Tofu can also be fried or baked. Tofu absorbs flavoring very well and can taste many ways depending how you season and cook it.

Tomatoes - Sliced cold tomatoes with red wine vinegar and ground peppercorn are a great side dish. Hot stewed tomatoes also make a good side dish.

Combination dishes

Beans & rice - Just mix and serve. Favorites are black beans, pinto beans, kidney beans and lima beans. Add some diced jalapeno pepper if you want to spice things up!

Beans & grains - Favorite grains are bulgur wheat, wheat berries, pearl barley, etc. Favorite beans are black eyed peas, black beans, pinto beans, kidney beans and lima beans.

Burritos - Burritos are a great alternative to sandwiches to take with you to lunch or on the road. It is hard to find store bought tortillas with good ingredients, instead make your own! There is a recipe for tortillas later in the chapter. Good ingredients for burritos are pinto beans, rice, spinach, stir fried bell peppers and onions, re-fried beans, black beans, avocado or guacamole, sauerkraut, shredded lettuce, etc.

Burrito bowls - Use the same ingredients as a burrito, but put it into a salad bowl without the tortilla.

Hot pots - A hot pot is a small pot or tall bowl that is used for each person. You start by filling your pot about half way with steaming hot soup stock, then you add ingredients of your choice to create your own custom soup or stew. The ingredients are served on common plates and are ready to be added to your hot pot. Some popular ingredients for traditional Asian hot pots are: rice, leaf vegetables, small pieces of meat, mushrooms, kombu, wakame, oysters and seafood. For customized hot pots you can have any ingredients that you would normally use for soup or stew.

Lentils & rice - Mix lentils and rice with curry powder or chili powder.

Sandwiches - Use real old world style whole grain bread if available, or bake your own bread. Almost all bread from grocery stores is way too processed, no matter what they claim on the label. See the bread recipes later in this chapter. Sandwiches are best when a compact higher energy meal is needed such as for hiking, cycling and other serious exercise.

- Nut butter and fruit sandwich - Any kind of reasonably dry fruit can be used such as sliced banana, mango, apple, pear, pineapple, etc.
- Avocado or guacamole and fruit sandwich - Any kind of reasonably dry tropical fruit can be used such as sliced bananas, mango, pineapple, etc.

- Avocado or guacamole and vegetable sandwich - Great with kale, cucumbers, tomato, lettuce, spinach, etc.

- Black bean patty sandwiches - Great with hummus, kale, spinach, bean sprouts, etc.

Vegetable rice - Any kind of vegetables can be mixed with rice and stir fried. Favorites are green peas, corn, chopped carrots, etc.

Wraps - Use a tortilla instead of bread to make any kind of sandwich that you like. The difference between a wrap and a burrito is that a wrap is usually served cold and has fresh green vegetables like a cold sandwich, a burrito is mostly made with cooked hot ingredients.

Recipes

Baked falafel - Falafel is the Middle Eastern equivalent of a hushpuppy (the deep fried cornbread balls, not the shoe!), but with much greater nutritional value. It is traditionally fried in oil, in this case we are baking it.

- 2 cups chickpeas, cooked, deshelled and drained (or canned).

- 1 cup chopped yellow onion.

- ¼ cup chopped green onion.

- 4 tablespoons ground flaxseed.

- 4 cloves diced garlic.

- 4 tablespoons almond butter or peanut butter.

- ¼ teaspoon coriander (ground or powder).

- ¼ teaspoon cumin (ground or powder).

- ¼ teaspoon chili pepper

- 1 tablespoon soy sauce

Puree all ingredients in a blender or food processor. Make into balls and place on a cookie tin or baking tin. Bake at 325 F to your preference.

Black bean patties - Black bean patties are great for sandwiches and as a side dish. They can also be cut up and added to salads and other dishes as an ingredient. This recipe is for basic black bean patties and can be modified by using different kinds of beans and seasonings. Black bean patties should be refrigerated or frozen for storage. The ingredients that follow will make 12 patties:

- 2 cans (15 oz size) black beans, drained and rinsed or a one pound package of dried black beans you have cooked. See chapter seven for cooking instructions for legumes.

- 1 cup whole grain flour or almond flour. Alternatively you can use bread crumbs.

- 6 tablespoons ground flaxseed.

- 6 cloves chopped garlic.

- 1 tablespoon lime rind (grated).

- 2 teaspoons chili powder.

- 1 tablespoon oregano.

- ½ teaspoon salt

- 1 cup chopped yellow onion (optional).

1. Optional step - spread the beans onto a baking pan and put them in the oven for 20 minutes at 325 F. This will make the patties drier and less mushy. Some people get better results with this step.

2. Mix all ingredients in a mixing bowl or use a power mixer.

3. Form the patties by hand and fry until firm. Black bean patties are more fragile than burgers so take care flipping and handling them.

Corn tortillas - Making corn tortillas requires fewer ingredients than flour tortillas, they are easy to make.

- 4 cups masa harina (hominy).

- 4 cups water.

- 1 teaspoon salt.

1. Mix all ingredients using a hand or power mixer.

2. Knead the dough for a few minutes.

3. Form balls of dough and use a rolling pin to flatten them into 10 inch diameter round tortillas (or whatever size you need).

4. Cook with a large skillet on medium-high, flip to cook both sides when ready.

Desi chickpea and okra patties - Desi chickpeas are nutty, dark brown and have far more texture than regular white chickpeas, even more than black beans. The ingredients that follow will make 12 patties:

- 1 pound of dried desi chickpeas (pre-cooked). See chapter seven for cooking instructions for legumes.

- 2 cups okra (frozen for fresh).

- 1 cup whole grain flour or almond flour. Alternatively you can use bread crumbs.

- 6 tablespoons ground flaxseed.

- 6 cloves chopped garlic.

- 1 tablespoon lime rind (grated).

- 2 teaspoons chili powder.
- 1 tablespoon oregano.
- ½ teaspoon salt
- 1 cup chopped yellow onion (optional).

Mix and chop the ingredients in a food processor. Form the patties by hand and fry until firm.

Dried kale - Dried kale can be eaten as a snack food or used as an ingredient in other dishes. The procedure below is done in a regular home oven and also works with other greens such as collard greens. Alternatively a food dehydrator can be used and will allow you to dehydrate much more at one time.

1. Boil chopped kale for 3 to 5 minutes, drain and cool.
2. Optionally season to taste with herbs and spices.
3. Place on an oven tin or other flat surface and allow to dry at room temperature or in an oven at a very low temperature such as 150 F.
4. When completely dry, optionally shred or break into smaller pieces.

Flour tortillas - Tortillas are a type of flatbread and are easy to make. Flour tortillas are made with wheat flour, but you can try other types of flour if you are adventurous. The ingredients for basic flour tortillas are as follows:

- 4 cups whole wheat flour (or other type of whole grain flour).
- 2 teaspoons salt.
- 4 tablespoons ground flaxseed.
- 2 tablespoons olive oil.
- 1 1/2 cups water (add more if needed).
- 2 tablespoons baking powder

1. Mix all ingredients using a hand or power mixer to make dough.
2. Knead the dough for a few minutes.
3. Form balls of dough and use a rolling pin to flatten them into 10 inch diameter round tortillas (or whatever size you need).
4. Cook with a large skillet on medium-high, flip to cook both sides when ready.

Hummus - This recipe is for basic hummus. You can add ingredients as desired to produce variations such as spicy hot hummus (add hot pepper), almond hummus (add almond butter), garlic hummus (add extra garlic or cubed garlic) or sun dried tomato hummus (add sun dried tomato pieces on top of the hummus).

The basic list of ingredients is as follows:

- 1 pound dried chickpeas (or 7 cups canned chickpeas).
- 1 cup tahini
- 1 cup lemon juice
- 12 cloves garlic, mashed
- ¼ cup olive oil (optional)
- ½ to 1 cup water (add until consistency is correct)
- 1 tablespoon salt
- 1 teaspoon fine ground black pepper

Cooking instructions are as follows:

1. If you are using 7 cups of canned chickpeas, drain the liquid and go to the next step. If you are using a one pound bag of dried chickpeas, put them in a pot and soak overnight if you have time, then boil for 5 minutes and simmer until tender. Without soaking, boil for 20 minutes then simmer until tender. You want the chickpeas tender enough that the skins start to come off. Rinse them in cold water and rub the skins off, you may need to rinse several times to get most of the skins off. Discard the skins and drain the water. If the skins won't come off they need more time simmering. If a few skins did not come off, that's OK, most of them should be off.

2. Depending on how big and powerful your food processor or blender is, you can make one large batch, or make several smaller batches. If you are not sure, make small batches, making larger batches of hummus can burn out lower power blenders and food processors because it is so thick.

3. If you are making one large batch, put the chickpeas from step 1 in the blender or food processor with all other ingredients except the water. If you are going to make 4 batches, divide the ingredients equally between the 4 batches. Add half only half the called for amount of water.

4. Run the food processor or blender until you get a smooth consistency. Add more water slowly if the mixture is too thick. Remember that you can always add water but you can't remove it if you add too much!

Oatmeal raisin cookies - This is a straightforward recipe for oatmeal cookies, you can substitute the raisins for another ingredient to make other types of oatmeal cookies. Some possible alternatives are almonds, dark chocolate chips, cubed dates, dried cranberries, dried mango pieces, peanuts, etc.

- 3 cups rolled oats.
- 1 cup whole grain stone ground flour.
- 1-½ cup raisins.

- 1 cup chopped walnuts.
- ½ cup soy or almond milk.
- 3/4 cup applesauce.
- 1/2 cup honey or turbinado sugar.
- 4 tablespoons ground flaxseed.
- ½ teaspoon baking soda.
- ½ teaspoon salt.
- 1 tablespoon molasses.
- 1-½ teaspoon vanilla extract.
- 1 tablespoon ceylon cinnamon.

Preparation and baking:

1. Mix ingredients by hand or use a power mixer.
2. Drop cookie sized spoons of cookie mix on a cookie sheet 2 or 3 inches apart.
3. Bake for 10 to 15 minutes (until lightly browned) at 325 F.

Potato, onion and spinach casserole - Bake at 325 F for 40 minutes.

- 4 cups sliced yellow onion.
- 3 cups sliced potato.
- 4 cups spinach.
- 1 pound sliced mushrooms.
- 1 cup of cooking wine.
- ½ cup ground soaked cashews.
- 4 cloves of minced garlic.
- ¼ cup chopped parsley.
- 1 teaspoon black pepper.
- 4 tablespoons ground flaxseed.
- 1/2 teaspoon sea salt.
- 2 cups cubed tofu (optional).

Soup - Soup is one of the easiest foods to make. Don't buy canned soup, almost all canned soup has processed ingredients and large amounts of salt. See the section "Making soup" in chapter seven for cooking instructions for soup. Preparing the soups below is a two step process. First, prepare the puree or stock. Second, add other ingredients and simmer until done. Some popular types of soup are listed below, the serving size is for 4 people (about 48 ounces of soup or 1-½ cups for each person).

- Tomato basil soup: Puree (in the blender): 2 pounds sliced tomatoes, 2 cups organic vegetable stock, 1 medium sized sliced yellow onion, 4 cloves mashed garlic, 2 cups fresh basil leaves, ½ teaspoon sea salt, 2 teaspoons chili powder, 1 spoon hot red pepper (optional). Simmer to taste. Sprinkle some basil leaves on top.

- Vegetable soup: Simmer 3 cups organic vegetable stock. Add 1 cup cubed potato, ½ cup chopped yellow onion, ½ cup cubed carrots, 1 cup cubed tomato, 4 cloves mashed garlic, ½ teaspoon sea salt, 1 teaspoon ground peppercorn.

- Split pea soup: Puree (in the blender): 3 cups of cooked split peas (see chapter seven for how to cook split peas), 1 cup chopped yellow onion, 3 cups organic vegetable stock, 2 cloves mashed garlic, ½ teaspoon sea salt, 2 teaspoons chili powder. Simmer to taste.

- Lentil soup: Puree (in the blender): 3 cups of cooked lentils (see chapter seven for how to cook lentils), 1 cup chopped yellow onion, 3 cups organic vegetable stock, 2 cloves mashed garlic, ½ teaspoon sea salt, 2 teaspoons curry powder, 1 spoon hot red pepper (optional). Simmer to taste.

- Cabbage soup: Simmer 4 cups organic vegetable stock. Add one pound of sliced cabbage, one large sliced yellow onion. Cook until the cabbage is tender. Do not drain. Season with red wine vinegar and ground peppercorn.

Stew - To make stew, start with making a thick puree in your blender. Some popular ingredients for the puree are tomatoes, sweet potato, pumpkin, lentils, split peas, white beans, rice, grains, etc. Alternatively you can used canned items such as diced tomato. After blending the puree, put it in a saucepan and let it simmer while you add additional pre-cooked ingredients such as corn, lima beans, carrots, cubed potato, cut green beans, lentils, chickpeas, etc. Season to taste and serve.

Tabbouleh - A Mediterranean salad. Preparation is easy, just mix everything together after preparing the bulgar wheat.

- 1 cup bulgur wheat (boil for 1 minute, let stand five minutes, drain).
- ¼ cup olive oil (or less).
- ½ cup lemon juice.
- 1 teaspoon sea salt.
- 2 teaspoons ground black peppercorn.
- 1 cup chopped parsley.
- ½ cup chopped red bell pepper.
- ½ teaspoon ground nutmeg.
- 3 cups chopped tomatoes.

- Flavored vinaigrette (optional).

Whole grain flaxseed bread - Basic bread recipe that makes 1 loaf. You can use any type of whole grain flour, the recipe is optimized for whole wheat. Use the following ingredients:

- 7 cups whole grain flour.
- 2 1/4 teaspoons, active dry yeast (2 packages).
- 2 cups warm soy or almond milk.
- 1 ¼ cup warm water.
- 1 ½ teaspoons (30 ml) salt.
- ½ cup ground flaxseed.
- 4 tablespoons honey.

1. Mix 1 cup warm water with 4 tablespoons of the honey, stir in the dry yeast. Let it sit until it is foamy.
2. Place all remaining ingredients in a mixing bowl with the yeast mixture and mix together.
3. Knead the dough for 3 to 5 minutes.
4. Let the dough rise for 2 hours in a warm place (or until it doubles in size).
5. Place the dough in a bread pan.
6. Bake 350°F for 45 minutes or until done.

Nut bread - Use the same recipe as whole grain flaxseed bread above, but add ½ cup of your favorites nuts such as; walnuts, almonds, peanuts, chia seeds, etc.

Beverages

Few drinks sold in stores are healthy. Dry tea is one exception, most types of tea sold in tea bags is very healthy. Most juice is processed and filtered with increased energy densities and should be avoided. Instead of buying drinks, you can make your own drinks with healthy ingredients. Smoothies are a great way to include fruit in your meals and they also good for appetizers. Using smoothies in this manner provides both a beverage and a couple portions of fruit or vegetables in your meal at the same time. Making smoothies is covered in chapter eight along with a type of sports drink called switchel.

Dessert

For dessert nature has already supplied a ready made solution, fruit! You can forever dispense with the refined and processed desserts from the American diet and eat a healthy fruit bowl instead, or just eat a piece of fruit. Alternatively a smoothie makes a great dessert. Making smoothies is covered in chapter eight.

Dressings & sauces

Most people think of salad when they think of dressing, but dressings and sauces can be used on many foods as a quick way to add flavor and substance. I think of dressings & sauces as the big equalizer that can help overcome complex seasoning problems. If you are seasoning something with herbs and spices and it is not coming out right, a quick save is to pour on some of your favorite dressing or sauce. The added volume of the dressing or sauce is often enough to mask whatever flavor malfunction was unfolding!

It is best to make your own dressings and sauces, most of the dressings and sauces sold in grocery stores are highly processed foods with many undesirable ingredients. It is easy to make dressings and sauces and far less expensive. You may have to go through some rounds of trial and error to get the exact taste you are looking for, but it will be worth it! If you are going to occasionally buy dressings and sauces, don't settle. Look closely at the list of ingredients.

Bottled sauces - Some of my favorite bottled sauces are salsa, applesauce, and some types of spaghetti sauce. Applesauce makes a great side dish when flavored with cinnamon.

Cooking wine - Cooking wine has a stronger taste than most regular drinking wine and has some extra salt and a higher alcohol content. This allows it to be used from an open bottle over a long period of time without going bad. Any inexpensive sweet red wine also works great for cooking. Try adding some cooking wine while stir frying or sauteing.

Creamy cashew sauce - To make cashew sauce, soak cashews in water or soy/almond milk overnight. Use a blender or food processor to puree them. Add water or soy/almond milk as needed to get the proper consistency. Use your choice of spices and seasonings such as curry powder, garlic, etc. To make the sauce lighter add some white beans (canned) while blending.

Flavored vinaigrette - This includes red wine vinegar, white wine vinegar, apple cider vinegar, balsamic vinegar, pepper vinegar, etc. You can make your own flavored vinegars by adding almost anything to vinegar. Add garlic cloves for garlic vinegar. Fruit vinegars and berry vinegars are great. Experiment, you really can't go wrong. Pour out some of the vinegar and add chopped or mashed spices, herbs or fruit. Let it age for a few days to several weeks. Write down what you did, so that if it's really good you can do it again. Seeds also work good, try fennel vinegar and sesame vinegar. Another idea is tahini vinegar or sesame oil vinegar.

Frozen orange or grape juice - Although frozen juice is not good to drink because of the processing and high energy density, it is great for flavoring food and as a sweetener, when compared to other sweeteners.

Hoisin sauce - Hoisin sauce is a type of Chinese barbecue sauce, traditionally made from toasted soybeans. Modern hoisin sauce is made from any of the following ingredients; sweet potato, wheat, rice, sugar, soybeans, white vinegar, salt, garlic, red chili pepper and sesame.

Hotsauce - There are many types of cayenne pepper based hot sauces. The flavoring for different brands varies greatly, try several to find your favorite. Some types are really hot, others are surprisingly mild but have a pronounced flavor.

Lemon or lime juice - You can squeeze your own or buy containers of lemon or lime juice.

Miso sauce - Miso is fermented soy that is used as a sauce or flavoring. Miso sauce can be purchased or made from miso powder. Miso powder can be found in Asian food stores or ordered online.

Molasses - With a strong flavor, molasses is the defining ingredient in many foods and drinks such as rum, dark beer, dark rye bread and many types of cookies. It is great as a syrup on pancakes and oatmeal.

Mustard - There are many types of mustard. Try different types until you find the type that you like.

Nut butters - Nut butters are best if you have access to a store with a grinder, so that you can grind them from fresh nuts. Most stores that have a bulk food department, have a grinder. Pre-made nut butter is ground too finely and may be many months old. You can also grind it yourself if you have a grinder. Some food processors can make nut butter, but make sure to read the manual or specifications for your processor, because nut butter is too thick and will burn out the motor on most food processors. Keep your eye on how much nut butter you eat, the stuff is almost addictive and it is easy to eat large quantities without realizing it.

Soy sauce - Soy sauce is probably the most popular Asian sauce and goes great on almost anything, it also makes a great ingredient. Don't overuse soy sauce however, it contains acrylamide, a known carcinogen. At some time in the future there may be a way to remove acrylamide from foods or produce an acrylamide free soy sauce, but in the mean time you should limit your consumption of soy sauce to occasional. Only buy naturally brewed soy sauce. Most major brands sold in the US are naturally brewed. The other method is chemically brewed, it is cheaper to make, but uses really nasty chemicals in the process that don't get fully removed.

Squash, pumpkin and sweet potato sauces - This includes pumpkin sauce. Canned pumpkin can be thinned and made into a sauce by adding water or soy/almond milk. Season with ceylon cinnamon and molasses. Squashes or sweet potato can be pureed in a blender or food processor, thinned by adding water or soy/almond milk and seasoned to taste.

Sriracha sauce - Sriracha sauce is a chili pepper hot sauce made from chili peppers, white vinegar, garlic, sugar and salt. It is popular for seafood but also is good on most other dishes. Because sriracha sauce is so hot, you won't use enough of it for the refined sugar to make any difference, or better yet, you can make it yourself.

Teriyaki sauce - Teriyaki sauce is a mixture of soy sauce, mirin (rice wine) and some type of sweetener. You can make your own teriyaki sauce easily.

Tomato sauce and tomato paste - Watch the ingredient list closely for tomato sauce, some brands try to slip in sugar, high fructose corn syrup or other unwanted ingredients.

Worcestershire sauce - Also called Worcester sauce it is a fermented vinegar sauce made with malt vinegar, molasses, anchovies, garlic, tamarind, onion and spices. It is hard to describe the taste, you just have to try some! Worcester sauce is great along with red wine when stir frying. It has an appearance similar to soy sauce, but more of a dark brown color.

Toppings & ingredients

Bread crumbs - Don't use the processed store bought kind, make your own from healthy whole grain European type bread. A food processor is good for this.

Chopped alliums - Chopped garlic, chopped onion, chopped leek, chopped green onion,

Chopped fennel bulb - The bulb of the fennel plant looks kind of like an onion but with a strong nutty flavor. You can cook it any of the ways that an onion can be cooked such as boiling, baking, frying. It can be used to flavor beans, lentils and many other dishes or you can eat it as a side dish by itself.

Chopped nuts - Almonds, walnuts, peanuts and cashews can be used on any dish. Use a blender or food processor to chop them or buy them chopped.

Cubed pineapple - Small freshly cut cubes of pineapple add a lot of flavor to almost any dish.

Dried mushrooms - For extra flavor and texture add chopped, dried mushrooms to soups, stews, beans, lentils, etc. Portobellos are milder, shiitake have a more pronounced flavor and texture.

Dried or roasted tomatoes - Slice and dry in the oven at 250 F for a couple hours. Try different sizes, temperatures and times until you get the right result. You can also buy dried tomatoes.

Nutritional yeast - Nutritional yeast has a great cheesy flavor.

Raisins & chopped dates - Raisins & chopped dates add a sweet chewy and fruity element to any dish even dishes like fried rice, beans, salads or soup.

Roast garlic - Roast garlic has a mild but distinctive flavor that is great on many types of food. Roast whole garlic at 325 F for 30 minutes, peel and mash. Make a lot at one time and then refrigerate in a sealed container.

Roast peppers - Roast peppers go great in salads and cooked dishes of all types. Cut the peppers up into strips and lay them out on an oven tray. Roast them in the oven for about an hour at 350 F.

Toasted seeds - You can buy toasted seeds or make your own. Set the oven for 300 F and toast for 5 to 10 minutes, shake them up several times during toasting. Toasted seeds add a lot of flavor to all types of dishes cooked greens to salads.

Herbs, spices & seasonings

In general, people's expectations for seasonings are high because of the chemical flavorings and high levels of salt used in the American diet. At first a whole food diet may seem bland, but with natural seasonings whole foods can taste better than the foods of the American diet. Whole foods have a stronger taste than processed foods and do not require the types of chemical seasoning and colorings used in processed foods.

It may take some time to become skilled at seasoning whole food. Don't add too many seasonings at the same time, it makes a disaster. Start with a little seasoning and add more gradually while you taste the food, you can always add more, but it is hard to remove seasoning!

Salt - As a general rule salt should not be added during cooking. Salt should be sprinkled on the surface of food when you are ready to eat, because salt on the surface of food has a much stronger taste than salt that is added during cooking. This allows you to use a much smaller quantity of salt for the same taste. Finely ground salt has a stronger taste than larger ground table salt. Sea salt also has a stronger taste. Sea salt is available in a grinder style container that produces very fine particle sizes. Make sure you regulate your total salt intake to the correct amount including the salt that is naturally in the food. This is covered in chapter four.

Substitutes for salt - Sea vegetables like kombu and wakame taste salty and can be used as a substitute for salt in some dishes such as seafood, fish and of course clam chowder. Lemon juice or seasonings with dried lemon like Mrs, Dash can also be used in many dishes instead of salt.

Herbs and spices - These are the herbs and spices that you actually want on hand because you will use them the most:

- Black pepper
- Ceylon cinnamon
- Coriander seed
- Cumin seed

- Curry powder
- Fennel seed
- Oregano
- Paprika
- Peppercorn (with grinder mill)
- Red pepper flakes
- Thyme
- Turmeric

Seasonings - These are the seasonings that you actually want on hand because you will use them the most:

- Chili mix
- Pinto bean seasoning
- Garlic Pepper
- Italian seasoning
- Kelp (seaweed)
- Lemon pepper
- Miso powder
- Mrs Dash (various salt free flavors)
- Season-All
- Taco seasoning
- Fajita seasoning

Buy when needed herbs and spices - In this category, buy only a small quantity when you actually need them. Herbs and spices lose their taste after a while and become worthless if they sit on the shelf too long.

Basil, Sage, Mint, Dill, Rosemary, Tea Leaf, Lavender, Ginger, Garlic powder, Allspice, Nutmeg, Ground cloves, Jalapeno pepper, Cayenne pepper, Parsley, Ground Onion, Alum, Bay leaves, Caraway seed, Mustard seed, Sesame seed, Saffron, Poppy seed, Anise seed, Arrowroot, ground garlic, ground onion.

Balanced lunch & dinner

Balanced meals consist of vegetables + fruits & berries + legumes + seeds & nuts + grains & starches. In the examples below, the portion size for the green vegetables like kale, collard greens and broccoli should be large, covering about half the plate. This is because green vegetables are low in calories so it takes a lot of them to make a balanced plate. The following are balanced lunch and dinner plates made from simple side dishes that go well together to form a balanced meal:

- Baked vegetables + Pineapple + Beans + Rice + Nut or seed topping.
- Kale + Asparagus + Bean salad + Mashed sweet potato + Nut or seed topping.
- Collard greens + Avocado + Lentils + Baked squash + Nut or seed topping.
- Steamed broccoli + Plantains + lima beans + Rice + Nut or seed topping.
- Brussels sprouts + Fruit smoothie + Split peas + Sweet potato + Nut or seed topping.
- Fruit bowl appetizer + Watercress + Lima beans + Yellow squash + Nut or seed topping.

Notice that in the last two examples a fruit bowl appetizer and a smoothie are used as the fruit & berry item. Another way to include fruit & berries is to have a piece of fruit for dessert, like an apple, peach or a bowl of grapes.

Creating a balanced plate that includes combos and recipes will look like the next examples:

- Vegetable/bean soup + Plantains + Falafel + Pearl barley/Chia seed + grapes.
- Burrito + Fruit & nut bowl.
- Tabbouleh + Potato, onion and spinach casserole + Fruit & nut bowl.

10 - Exercise & Fitness

In the first part of this chapter we will cover exercise, in the second part, nutrition for exercise and sports.

Many Americans don't exercise. Americans that exercise tend to do periodic "workouts". Doing a workout is usually viewed as a chore and normally consists of a 20 to 40 minute period of semi-intense exercise every other day or three times a week. Although this is better than no activity at all, sporadic workouts do not result in a high level of fitness. These workouts don't feel good. Most people dread having to face their workouts. Cycles of inactivity are common when other more important activities get in the way.

If we look at history to determine what is normal and healthy for humans in regard to exercise, we find that the human body is designed to be in motion during most of our waking hours. The modern sedentary lifestyle is not normal or healthy.

Exercise throughout the day

We should exercise throughout the day, like our ancestors did. We should stay as active as possible and do some form of exercise about every two hours, even if its just walking for five or ten minutes. You should exercise at least 60 minutes every day, and preferably for 90 minutes or more. You are probably thinking that you don't have the time to exercise for 60 minutes a day, so we will address the time issue in the next section. Daily exercise should be a combination of activities. For example:

- 7AM   Run or walk to the store for 20 minutes.
- 9AM   Walk 5 minutes.
- 10AM Do bodyweight exercises for 10 minutes.
- 12PM Jump rope and do pushups for 5 minutes.
- 2PM   Walk or run up and down stairs for 5 minutes.
- 4PM   Run around the parking lot for 5 minutes.
- 6PM   More walking.
- 8PM   Take a bike ride for 30 minutes with high intensity intervals.

As you can see, individually these activities are trivial, nothing to dread. In fact they are fun and will make you feel good. Exercising throughout the day, you will total a lot of activity. The goal is to break from a sedentary routine and keep moving. You should do a variety of exercises. It is important that they are fun, so you will look forward to them and will continue to do them as a continuous part of your daily life. Break free from the mindset in which exercise consists of some period of intense and dreaded activity, after which you are done. Your body needs activity throughout the day.

Longer periods of more intense exercise can be done in the early morning or evening so that it will be convenient to shower if needed. Shorter periods of exercise can be interspersed with your work day, school day or whatever you do. The shorter periods of exercise can be done in whatever clothes you are wearing, and will not generate enough sweat to be an issue, you will cool down relatively quickly.

If you watch a lot of television you can exercise during commercial breaks. With the ever increasing amount of commercials that are shown, some commercial breaks can be over 3 minutes long. It is possible to do a lot of exercise during these breaks. Another option is to use an exercise bike or rowing machine while you are watching television.

If you are lucky, you work in a job that keeps you on your feet and moving most of the time. In this case you may want to do additional exercise in the early mornings or evenings, but a substantial part of your exercise can be done at work. Jobs like waiting tables are real exercise, using a pedometer to track the distance covered, you will find that the average waiter or waitress can cover 5 to 10 miles a day.

Yes, but I don't have the time

The time spent doing exercise is not lost, much of it is made up through increased productivity. Countless studies have shown that exercise makes people more productive. There are many reasons for this. Blood circulation increases nutrients and oxygen to the brain. Exercise increases brain activity (to coordinate motor function). Exercise increases health.

The average American spends over 5 hours a day watching television, 30 additional minutes watching recorded television, 1 hour on a home computer and over 1 hour using a smartphone. That totals 8 hours or more per day using electronic devices outside of work. As a matter of priorities, some time can be shifted from using electronic devices and spent getting exercise.

Some types of exercise can be combined with other tasks. For example you can walk, run or bicycle to the store (or other places) instead of driving a car. This may even save time if there is traffic. An example of exercise combined with work is digging in the vegetable garden or building something. Another example is talking on the phone while walking.

Time can be saved by reducing or eliminating forms of exercise with high overhead such as going to the gym. Going to the gym typically involves changing clothes, getting in a car and driving, waiting for equipment, unwanted social interaction, etc. Your exercise regimen should be structured around forms of exercise with low overhead. An example of low overhead exercise is walking or running, this can be done anywhere with little or no preparation.

The role of exercise in weight loss

Weight loss is 80% or 90% dominated by your diet. Think of exercise as the helper and your diet as the main actor that will drive weight loss. Exercise is very important to your health and will speed up weight loss dramatically, but without a good diet it is difficult to lose weight or maintain a healthy weight, no matter how much exercise you do. An example of this is a new demographic category called the "fat fit" that companies are developing and marketing products for. These people exercise for hours a day and are still overweight.

Forms of exercise

Basic forms of exercise should comprise the foundation of your long term exercise routine. This is important, because this puts you in total control of your exercise schedule and means that you can adjust your exercise routine as unexpected events take place, instead of putting your routine on hold. You can do most forms of basic exercise anywhere and at any time.

Walking and hiking

Walking is a serious form of exercise, many people walk as their only form of exercise and remain in great shape. Aggressive walking, walking uphill or walking with weight, can have the same aerobic and cardio benefits as jogging or running with lower stress on the body. Although stress is not an issue with most people (and can even be beneficial), some people with bone or joint issues find that the reduced stress of walking can be an advantage.

Jogging and running

Jogging and running complement walking, combined they make a great workout with varying intensities. Walking can be done for the warm-up and cool down phase with intervals of jogging, running and walking in between. This never gets boring. You can run or jog as long as it feels good and then slow to a walk until you are ready to run or jog again. Starting out, some people only run a few hundred feet at a time, but over time this will increase. I know people who are running distances now that never thought they could run again. This type of unstructured exercise is much more enjoyable than a forced routine, and you are more likely to adopt this as a permanent part of your life for many years to come. Even athletes can benefit from listening to their bodies and being a little less structured in their routines.

Many people that have joint issues associated with running find that these issues are caused by bad running form and poor footwear. Changing to flat footwear and a forefoot/mid-foot strike instead of a heel strike can eliminate joint and impact issues. Adopting flatter footwear may seem counter-intuitive, but modern wedge shaped running shoes with lots of cushioning in the heel promote a heel strike running style that can injure ankle, knee, hip and spinal joints. This is because the motor feedback functions of the brain sense the extra cushioning and adjust your running form to favor a heel strike. To illustrate this, try taking off your shoes and running barefoot on a hard surface like asphalt or cement. Your brain will automatically adjust your form to a forefoot/mid-foot strike to compensate for the lack of cushioning. The reverse happens when you add cushioning, your brain senses the cushioning and adjusts your form to favor a heel strike.

When you run with a heel strike you are depending on the cushioning of the shoe, your body does not provide much natural cushioning in the heel. Actually your body is designed to provide enough cushioning for walking with a heel strike (which is natural), but not for running. With a forefoot/mid-foot strike the muscles and tendons of your foot and lower leg provide spring force and cushioning that is far greater than the cushioning that can be provided by a shoe, even if it had inches of cushioning. This is the issue that is driving the current barefoot running craze, but although barefoot running can have advantages, it takes time to build up the required foot strength. Most of the benefit of barefoot running can be had by using a forefoot/mid-foot strike with low profile (flat) footwear, and the wear and tear on the feet is much less than running barefoot.

Switching to a forefoot/mid-foot strike should be done little by little over a long time period (six months to a year) to allow the required muscle and tendon strength to develop. If a heel strike runner abruptly changes form and runs with a forefoot/mid-foot strike, they may damage their achilles tendon and possibly other tendons, muscles and connective tissue.

Many runners, particularly runners with flat feet, think that they need the support of highly cushioned shoes or even arch supports. Actually the opposite is the case. Highly cushioned shoes cause a reduction of muscle strength as the feet rely more and more on the cushioning of the shoe. As the feet become weaker, most people compensate by buying shoes with additional cushioning. As this vicious cycle continues, the feet become weaker and weaker until the arch becomes no longer able to support itself. The answer is the reverse of problem. Build the muscles of the feet by removing the cushioning and may be uncomfortable. It should be done little by little. Try wearing flat footwear with no arch support until it becomes painful, then cycle back to cushioned footwear and let your feet recover. Cycle back and forth as needed as your feet build strength, one day you can throw the cushioned footwear and arch supports in the trash!

Bicycling

Bicycling can provide more cardio benefits with less stress than most other forms of exercise except swimming and rowing. This is because of the smooth and continuous motion of the crank and pedals. Bicycling is a great exercise to alternate with walking and running. You can alternate days between bicycling and running (or walking). Some people do most of their biking in the summer and walk and run more in the winter.

In most weather and especially in hot weather, it is easier to achieve higher levels of cardio activity on a bicycle without an intense and concerted effort. There are several reasons for this. Bicycling is done at higher speeds, the airflow helps you stay cooler and feeling better. The higher speeds are fun and keep your mind occupied with navigation instead of thinking about every step. The rotary motion of the pedals is continuous and it is easier to go into "autopilot" on a bike. After a while you can forget that you are the one supplying the energy, you will just pedal automatically. This state of mind is more difficult for most people to attain while running.

Bicycling makes a good alternative to cars for local transportation. For short trips of under five miles (or even longer if there is traffic) you may find that a bicycle is faster than a car. Different routes and shortcuts are often possible with a bicycle. Parking is not a concern in most places with a bicycle.

If you are only using a bike for exercise or short trips, think about getting a relatively inexpensive and heavy clunker like a mountain bike or cross bike. This will allow you to get more exercise while traveling a shorter distance. Riding on bike trails and sidewalks gets you off the street and makes for a more pleasant ride, in which you will not be breathing large quantities of automobile exhaust or spending your entire ride tracking cars as they whiz by you at high speed. A road bike is too fast to get meaningful exercise riding in this manner and is too fragile to comfortably ride on trails and sidewalks.

If you prefer a road bike and wish to travel longer distances, you can ride on the road with little or no interference from cars by riding late at night or very early in the morning. Most cities have bike clubs that go out at these times. Having multiple riders increases safety and awareness of car traffic. Because there is less traffic late at night or very early in the morning, you will be breathing far less automobile exhaust. Many people have two bikes, a clunker for local rides on trails and a road bike for longer distance riding on the road.

Swimming

Water resistance exercise offers an excellent cardio workout with low overall stress. Different muscle groups are used then in other exercises, so swimming makes a good complement to other forms of exercise. Swimming works well for overweight or injured people, the stress level is far lower than any other type of exercise, because the weight is supported by the water.

Strength training

Strength training includes resistance exercises, crossfit, yoga, pilates, body weight exercises and weightlifting. These types of exercises can be done individually or in a scheduled group. The most beneficial forms of strength training are compound types of exercise that utilize multiple muscle groups at the same time, such as crossfit, yoga and pilates. Resistance training and weight lifting can use compound exercises, but often single muscle groups are targeted. Some types of strength training such as crossfit have aerobic components that increase both strength and cardiovascular fitness.

When lifting weights or working with resistance, medium or high numbers of repetitions at less than your maximum weight capacity are good. This goes against common practice in most weight lifting programs. Higher repetitions at a lower weight place far less stress on tendons and joints, but are still very beneficial and will build muscle mass. Higher reps also introduce a cardio component. The reason why most weight lifting programs stress using low reps at high weight is that the sets can be done faster and it is slightly more effective at building muscle mass, but at the cost of developing joint problems. Building muscle mass at a slightly lower rate but remaining free of injuries makes sense.

Exercise machines

Exercise machines such as treadmills or exercise bikes can provide a cardio workout when outdoor conditions prevent other forms of exercise, or when staying in hotels. Exercise machines should not be relied on as a primary means of exercise, because people rarely continue a regimen of machine exercise for more than a year. Machines may provide a workout, but they quickly become boring. Long term exercise must be fun or you won't continue.

Rowing machines like the Concept2 machines are somewhat expensive, but are far more beneficial than treadmills or exercise bikes. This is because rowing machines provide a fantastic cardio workout while building several muscle groups. Its like doing back, arm and leg exercises and getting a cardio workout all at the same time. Rowing makes it easier to sustain a more intense cardio workout then a treadmill or exercise bike can provide with the same perceived effort. This is because more muscle groups are being used at the same time.

Scheduled or group exercise

Scheduled or group exercise generally require other people or facilities and are usually done at a scheduled time. Some types of group exercise can be practiced individually if you have the equipment or facilities available. Some examples of scheduled exercise that can be integrated into your routine are: crossfit, gym workouts, cycling clubs, sports (basketball, soccer, track, etc), hiking trips, swimming, tennis, golf, martial arts, skiing, dance, etc. Scheduled or group exercise can be part of your exercise regimen but should not be relied on for your entire regimen, because exercise should be distributed throughout the day.

Do a variety of exercises

It is important to engage in a variety of exercise. Doing a variety of exercise works different muscle groups. This is similar to your diet, where eating a variety of food gives you the best results. People tend to fixate on one type of exercise at the exclusion of everything else. The problem comes when they can't perform their chosen exercise for some reason, such as boredom, soreness or injury, bad weather, end of the season, change of weather, vacation, holidays, etc. They tend to stop exercising. With a variety of exercises there will always be something fun you can do.

Challenge yourself

Some part of your exercises should be challenging, you should push yourself. The goal is to intermittently exercise with an increased intensity level that will cause high exertion (controlled stress). Your body reacts to muscle stress by building new muscle. Bone stress causes bone density to increase. Controlled stress is not the same thing as damage. Learn the difference between a controlled level of stress and damage. An example of controlled stress is when you have a hard workout and your muscles get sore.

We have already talked about diet related reasons for bone density loss, lack of exercise also causes bone density loss. Exercise and activity builds bone density. This is a normal body function. To illustrate, look what happens when astronauts spend time in space with no gravity, in as little as 90 days they will lose ten percent or more of their bone density. This is because the bones are not being stressed (flexing, compression, etc) as the muscles are used to counteract gravity during exercise and normal daily activity. The body is programmed to remove unneeded bone density. If there is little or no stress the body interprets this to mean that the bone density is unneeded and the body removes the unneeded bone material. On the other hand under the earth's normal gravity the bones must carry your weight and are under constant stress, this causes your body to maintain your bone density. Increased activity causes increased stress and bone density will increase.

The same holds true for muscle mass. With decreased use (like if you are sedentary or when astronauts are in space) the muscles will naturally atrophy at an alarming rate. This is a cruel fact of life. It can take years to build a perfect physique with strong muscles, but a relatively short period of inactivity will destroy most of the hard work. On the other hand your body does offer you a great deal. For every weak muscle cell you damage or kill, your body will replace it with one or more strong cells. When you challenge your body and put your muscles under controlled stress you cause weak muscle cells to be replaced by new strong cells and more cells to be added.

Training for events (real or unknown) is a great way to add purpose and intensity to your exercise routine. Pick some event in the future, like a particular hike, run or long bicycle riding event. Train for this event. Many times you can convince other people into committing to an event, people love a challenge, and then you can train together. This is a great way to get people involved in exercise that don't have the discipline otherwise. When I said unknown events I wasn't trying to be funny. I have met some preppers (people who believe and prepare for doomsday scenarios) who are constantly training and are in excellent physical condition. An unknown but possible event on the horizon gives them a purpose and reason to exercise at a level that they otherwise would probably not be able to achieve.

Intensity

It is best to exercise at varying levels of intensity. When you have a lot of energy, do more intense exercise, when you feel tired go slower. Listen to your body and let your body guide you. This creates an exercise regimen that is sustainable and will become an integral and permanent part of your life. Forcing intense workouts into a compressed timeframe feels bad and will not result in a permanent regimen, you will soon grow to hate it and quit. The most important thing is to get out of the house and exercise frequently. Some days you won't feel like exercising. Walk out the door anyway and walk down the street for a ways. If you still don't feel it, I go back home and try again later, but most of the time once you are out the door your mood will change and you will want to keep going.

High intensity interval training

HIIT stands for High Intensity Interval Training. A typical HIIT workout consists of a 10 minute warm-up and then brief periods of intense exertion followed by reset periods of lower exertion, followed by a cool down. The intense exertion periods last from 20 seconds to 2 minutes each and the reset periods typically last 5 minutes or less. There are from 3 to 6 high-intensity/reset cycles in most HIIT workouts. A HIIT workout will have the same cardio and muscle building benefit as a much longer period of normal exercise.

HIIT can be applied to running, bicycling, swimming and even strength training. Any type of exercise that can be done at a high level of exertion can be done as a HIIT workout. A HIIT running workout can consist of jogging for 10 minutes followed by high intensity intervals of sprinting at near top speed followed by reset periods of jogging at low speed. I like to incorporate 4 or 5 HIIT cycles at the end of a long bike ride, walk or run because I am already fully warmed up and ready to get home, the HIIT workout makes an exciting ending.

If you have not previously done HIIT workouts, be sure to work up to high intensity over a period of time, this may take several months, depending on your condition. This is to let your body build up to this type of activity and to prevent injury. Keep in mind that "high intensity" means high intensity for you, everyone is at a different level of physical fitness and the goal of a HIIT workout is to promote positive health, not to go beyond "high intensity" and cross the line into "damaging intensity". For sedentary or obese people high intensity may be a fast walk for 20 seconds interspersed with reset periods of very slow walking. If you are not sure about your physical condition or have health issues, see your doctor before engaging in HIIT. There are links to more info about HIIT in chapter twelve.

Breaking the rules

Stretching - Stretching is optional. For normal exercise it is not mandatory to stretch. You should stretch when it feels good. Of course if you are in competition sports it would be a good idea to stretch before doing explosive exercises like sprinting. Stretching can also be used to increase your range of motion or as a low intensity form of exercise. Stretching your calves one or two times a week can be used to avoid painful leg cramps (also known as a charley horse).

Exercise any time - There is no wrong time to exercise. It is OK to exercise at almost anytime, including before bed. Exercise before bed does not interfere with sleep, it is actually the opposite. Exercise makes you tired and it is easier to go to sleep. A warm up should be done if you have been sedentary for a long time to give your circulation a chance to increase, and of course strenuous exercise should be avoided right after a meal to allow your food time to digest. Other than that, exercise at any time! Some people will point out the exercising raises the metabolism and it is beneficial to do this in the morning, but this really does not make a big difference. Exercising when it fits your schedule will cause you to exercise more, this has a far greater impact on your health than the time of day in which you exercise.

Getting sleep & reducing stress

Sleep - Getting proper sleep is essential to good health. Insufficient sleep weakens the immune system and increases susceptibility to disease. Lack of sleep has a profound negative effect on productivity and cognitive ability. The proper amount of sleep for adults is at least 7-½ hours to 8-½ hours. Proper amounts of sleep correlate to maximum productivity and brain function. Sleep can be broken into two four hour blocks with a one or two hour waking period in the middle of the night. Historically this was the sleep pattern for most humans before the modern era.

Some people have a habit of chronically getting insufficient sleep. They are convinced that they are different from other people and do not need as much sleep (or are not able to get as much sleep for some reason). It is extremely rare for this to be caused by a medical condition. The cause is usually one of the following:

- Bad sleep habits. People tend to do what they are used to doing. Bad habits can be broken and replaced by good habits. Force yourself into good sleep schedule and it will become habit in a short time.

- The belief that higher productivity comes from working more hours and getting less sleep.

- Interference from stimulants (like caffeine), chemicals or drugs. Identify and eliminate anything that is interfering with your natural sleep cycle.

- Sedentary lifestyle. Lack of exercise can wreak havoc on your sleep cycle. Your body is designed to be in motion. Being sedentary causes many body functions to go off schedule, sleep is just one of them.

Stress - Exercise is one of the most powerful stress relievers known. If you suffer from stress, use exercise as your primary weapon. Exercise is a healthy way to control stress instead of drugs or alcohol. Getting the proper amount of sleep will also help reduce and control stress.

Nutrition for exercise and sports

This section covers nutritional concerns specific to exercise and sports.

Gaining muscle mass:

If you want to build muscle mass, you must work out. There is no other way to gain muscle mass except for enhancement drugs, which are a very bad idea because they have serious side effects and health risks. You can not build muscle mass by eating. This includes eating large amounts of protein. You do need a nutritionally adequate amount of protein in your diet, but additional protein will not give you added muscle mass. That would be like eating brains to get smarter, it just doesn't work that way. Eating too much fat and sugar will make you fat, but eating extra protein does not build muscle mass. This is explained in detail in the next section.

Protein

Selling protein is big business. Entire industries such as the meat, dairy and supplement industries are built on selling protein. Marketing protein is done by making people believe that high levels of protein are vital and beneficial. This type of marketing has been going on for over fifty years and has been very effective at establishing a perceived need for products that are high in protein. The idea that more protein is better has been promoted so heavily, that by now it is commonly accepted by most people as a fact.

In athletics the idea is promoted that protein somehow "feeds" muscles and that hard workouts or serious bodybuilding require large amounts of protein, the more the better. Most athletes have this understanding and will point out that this can't be wrong because everyone seems to agree. This idea is so well established that most athletes think they "need" extra protein or they will become fatigued.

In reality protein is like any other nutrient, you need the right amount to facilitate proper body function. Too little will cause a deficiency and too much will cause unwanted complications and side effects. According to the WHO (World Health Organization) the protein requirement for most humans is .83 grams of protein per 1 kilogram of body weight (.38 grams per pound). This equals about 56 grams of protein for a 150 pound man and 46 grams of protein for a 120 pound woman. The WHO requirement is substantially above the deficiency level, which means that there is a substantial safety margin built in. The USDA Reference Dietary Intake (RDI) is essentially the same as the WHO requirement. A balanced whole food diet will exceed the WHO and RDI recommendations.

Protein can't be stored by the body. Any protein that is not used by the body is burned as energy. Think of it like a coffee cup. To fill the cup you need a certain amount of coffee. Extra coffee that is poured in just spills over, the cup does not have the means to store extra coffee. There is no benefit to pouring in extra coffee, in fact there are unintended negative consequences like messing up the floor. This is similar to the situation with protein, except the negative consequences of too much protein are more severe than spilled coffee.

Protein is not the best source of energy for the human body, carbohydrates are the preferred source. This is because the body must do an extra conversion when using protein as a source of energy that is not required with carbohydrates. This conversion taxes the liver and other organs and is less efficient than using energy directly from carbohydrates. Additionally, the catabolic processing of protein (the reduction of protein to energy), increases acid levels in the bloodstream. The body uses calcium from the bones to neutralize this unwanted acid. This causes a loss of bone density and can result in brittle bones and osteoporosis later in life. High levels of protein increase levels of Insulin-like growth factor 1 (IGF-1) which promote cancer and other diseases. IGF-1 also significantly contributes to rapid aging. Sufficient protein should be consumed to support the anabolic processes (building of muscles and tissue), but large amounts of additional protein should be avoided.

But what about the increased protein needs of athletes? The idea that athletes have increased protein requirements or will benefit from increased protein consumption is a widely held misconception that is not supported by peer reviewed scientific research. Building muscles and connective tissue cells happens slowly over a period of time. The digestive system breaks down protein into amino acid components which travel through the bloodstream and are eventually assembled into muscle cells where they are needed. That's why it takes time to build muscle. Think about it, if the protein that you ate went immediately to your muscles you would be able to build huge muscles in a few days by eating lots of protein. Obviously that doesn't happen!

In fact there are no peer reviewed scientific studies showing a benefit from extra protein when the WHO requirements are used as a baseline. Additional calories that are consumed to supply energy for prolonged high level exertion have the same protein percentages as the baseline diet. What this means is that athletes may consume more energy than the baseline of approximately 2300 calories to compensate for prolonged athletic activity and that the percentage of protein consumed as part of the additional calories will be approximately the same as what is in the baseline diet. The information commonly cited by companies selling protein products and by sports nutritionists recommending high protein consumption are not peer reviewed science, they are usually misrepresentations of research that is taken out of context or are anecdotal in nature.

The bottom line is that the WHO and USDA RDI recommended protein intake is more than enough for any athlete, including weight lifters. Extra protein or protein supplements are not required or beneficial. If you are doing strenuous activities for prolonged periods of time you will naturally eat more food and therefore will get some additional protein from that additional food. This is more than enough to take care of your body's protein requirements for strenuous exercise and training. A balanced whole food diet will easily exceed the protein requirements of athletes without the consumption of supplements, meat or other types of animal products.

Carbohydrates

In a whole food diet most of your energy will come from carbohydrates. If you feel that you need to boost your short term energy level, eat some fruit. Bananas are great for this because they are high in potassium. Avoid refined carbohydrates (also known as simple carbohydrates), such as sugar, processed foods and processed drinks including energy drinks and sports drinks (see the sections below on water and salt). The complex carbohydrates in whole foods provide better long term energy and don't cause nausea and sugar rushes.

Fats

Fat is the primary source of long term energy and is also used by your body for storing energy. In most shorter athletic events you will burn carbohydrates, fat burning does not take place until your body runs out of carbohydrates to burn.

Water

There is no need to use sports drinks, the refined sugar and other processed ingredients in sports drinks are not healthy or needed. The only ingredient in sports drinks that you may need during extended strenuous exercise is salt, and this is covered in the next section. The marketing hype from sports drink suppliers about electrolytes are scientific tidbits cited out of context to sound impressive and sell products. If you are doing strenuous exercise and require extra salt, just add the correct amount of salt to your water instead of buying sports drinks.

If you don't like drinking plain water, consider putting a squirt of lemon juice in your water or making switchel. Switchel is a sports or hot weather drink made from water, vinegar and ginger. Some people add lemon juice, salt or molasses.

In hot climates while doing strenuous exercise sweat loss can be in the range of .5 to 1.2 liters per hour for most people in good physical condition. Make sure to remain hydrated but not over-hydrated. Dehydration can lead to injuries, especially in hot climates. Over-hydration can lead to hyponatremia. In general if your urine is a dark color and urination is infrequent and low in volume, you need to increase your consumption of water. If urination is frequent with high volume, and the color of your urine is clear you should cut back on water consumption.

Salt

For strenuous exercise lasting less than 1-½ hours or moderate exercise lasting less than 3 hours, normal dietary sodium intake is sufficient. For strenuous exercise lasting more than 1-½ hours particularly at high temperatures or when sweating heavily for long periods of time, iodized table salt should be added to your drinking water at the rate of ¼ teaspoon per liter. Table salt is about 40% sodium, so this is equal to 575 mg of sodium added per liter. The rate of sodium loss in physically fit people ranges from 500 mg to 1100 mg per liter of sweat. The replacement rate is not on a one to one basis because more water will be consumed than the amount of sweat that is lost. For more information there is a military technical bulletin that goes into great detail about salt and hydration requirements for strenuous exercise and exercise in extreme hot weather, links to the bulletin are in chapter twelve.

Supplements

Throw your supplements in the trash. Supplements are dangerous and cause twenty percent of all liver damage in the United States. The supplement industry is largely unregulated, and the United States government shows little interest getting it under control. Don't make supplement suppliers rich at your expense, save your money. There is no benefit to taking supplements when you are on a whole food diet because a whole food diet already supplies more than enough of everything your body needs. For many thousands of years people ate a whole food diet without supplements. Supplements are a processed product made in a factory. There is nothing natural about supplements despite what the labels and marketing may say.

Frequently Asked Questions

Question: What about structured exercise programs like the ones offered on DVD that I see on TV?

Answer: There are many structured exercise programs that are marketed, most of them targeted on weight loss, or perfect sculpted bodies. Almost everyone has several sets of exercise DVD's or books gathering dust. These programs promise big results but rarely deliver. If you like to do structured exercise programs intermittently that's fine, but a good permanent exercise regimen will always be founded on a variety of activities that can be done anywhere and anytime such as walking, running, biking, etc. There are some of these programs that offer a good selection of exercises. If you find a good program that you like, you can incorporate it as a part of your exercise regimen.

11 - Nutrition Software

This chapter is optional reading and covers nutritional analysis software and food composition data that can be used to evaluate food or plan your diet. As we talked about in chapter four, you do not need to use nutritional software to have a balanced whole food diet. If you follow the section "Balanced breakfast" at the end of chapter eight and the section "Balanced lunch & dinner" at the end of chapter nine, you will automatically have a balanced diet.

Nutritional analysis software

Nutritional analysis software is used to calculate the amount of nutrients in your food, including both macronutrients and micronutrients. The following are some examples of ways that nutritional analysis software can be used:

- Dietary planning and optimization.
- Tracking nutrient intake for medical analysis.
- Fine tuning nutrient intake during intense athletic training.
- Identifying nutritional deficiencies.
- Isolating food allergies.
- Keeping a record of diet and nutrition.

Nutritional analysis software should not be confused with simple diet software or label scanning apps for smart phones that track fat, carbohydrates and protein for the purpose of counting calories and dieting. Diet software and label scanning apps serve no purpose with a balanced whole food diet, because your body will automatically regulate your food intake and counting calories or keeping track of fat, carbohydrates and protein is unnecessary.

Your meals are entered into nutritional analysis software by looking up each ingredient using a database of foods (food composition data). After the meals are entered, the software calculates the total nutritional value of the meals. This can be done for individual meals and recipes, or for all meals in a day or all meals in a longer period of time like a week or month. Entering meals, ingredient by ingredient is tedious, but most software allows you to save and recall meals and recipes, so this only needs to be done once. After your favorite meals are entered and saved, you can simply recall them to make your meal plans.

There are two types of nutritional analysis software, cloud based and stand alone. Cloud based software uses a web browser or a smartphone interface, you must be connected to the Internet to use it. Stand alone software runs on a PC or Mac and does not require an Internet connection.

Food composition data

Nutritional analysis software gets its information about food from a food composition database. A typical food composition database lists thousands of foods and the nutrients they contain, including the macronutrients and micronutrients. Creating a food composition database is very expensive and is usually done at the government level. Several countries make databases available as a public service.

- The USDA National Nutrient Database for Standard Reference is compiled by the US Department of Agriculture and is probably the most used nutritional database. It is updated about once a year and includes 150 nutrients quantities for 8618 foods. It is available for download in several formats, but most nutritional software already includes the database, so it is usually not necessary to download it separately unless you need the raw data. It is also available in an online searchable version.

- The European Food Information Resource Network works to standardize food composition databases from European countries (and some other countries) and maintains a list of databases from member countries that are available online or for download. Member countries include Germany, Denmark, Italy, UK, France, Spain, Canada, Austria, Poland and about 60 others.

In addition to supplying the data for nutritional analysis software, food composition data can be used directly. An example is to compare the nutritional value of different foods or compare raw foods to cooked foods of the same type to understand the nutritional losses or gains caused by cooking. Surprisingly, some foods increase in nutritional value when cooked because trapped nutrients are made bioavailable by chemical changes that take place in the food when heated.

Food composition databases

- USDA Food composition databases - http://www.ars.usda.gov/Services/docs.htm?docid=8964
- USDA Food composition databases - http://www.ars.usda.gov/Services/docs.htm?docid=24912
- European Food Information Resource Network - http://www.eurofir.org/?page_id=96

Free software VS paid software

Nutritional analysis software comes in free and paid versions. There are good examples of both. Most of the free versions are web based, open source or sponsored by government organizations. Most nutritional analysis software uses the USDA database or one of the European databases (or data from multiple sources). Some of the paid software vendors claim they use a modified or cleaned database, but I have found little difference between the raw data from the government agencies and the databases used in paid software.

If you are interested in using nutritional analysis software I recommend that you first try free software, it may fill your needs. Some paid versions have a free trial, this will allow you to test before you buy. There are some very expensive software packages that are used by nutritionists, the difference is primarily the graphics presentation and added features such as the inclusion of supplements in the database (which is not needed with a whole food diet) and contact management so that nutritional practitioners can track their clients. Some of the paid software packages are able to generate impressive looking charts and graphs.

Web based nutritional software

SuperTracker (https://www.supertracker.usda.gov) - Supertracker is from the USDA and is web browser based. It has many features such as the ability to create accounts, multiple profiles, build recipes, combos and meals, look up foods, run reports, track physical activity, set goals and even keep a journal. This site is under constant development and is getting quite sophisticated, it may be all you need and best of all it's is free. Because it is web based you can access it through any computer. SuperTracker seems to work fine with newer smartphones running the Chrome web browser.

Cronometer (https://cronometer.com) - Cronometer has a free web version and paid apps ($2.99) for Android and iOS that let you access your account from a smartphone. The free web based version is easier to use and faster than Supertracker with many of the same features. There is a paid premium upgrade available for the web version, but the free version has enough features for most people and may be all you need.

DTU Food (http://www.foodcomp.dk/v7/fcdb_search.asp) - This simple online database tool from the Technical University of Denmark lets you look up any food and see the nutritional breakdown. It has a fast interface and no login required.

PC, Linux and Mac based nutritional software

Cronometer (Windows version http://cronometer.com/download/) - This is a stand alone version similar to the web based above, but will run with no Internet connection on computers with Windows. Also runs on Linux systems by using Wine.

Nut Nutrition (http://sourceforge.net/projects/nut/?source=recommended) - This open source software runs under TCL/TC/SqlLite on Windows, Linux or Mac systems. Because it is open source you can modify it, if you know how to program computers.

NutriSurvey - (http://www.nutrisurvey.de/) - This is an English translation of the commercial German EBISpro software that is free to download for non commercial use.

This software was written for diet assessment of populations and has some interesting features. It runs on Windows systems.

Android and iPhone

The Android and iPhone based nutritional software I have seen so far has not been very impressive, but this is a rapidly changing market and there may be apps that I have missed. One solution is to access the web based nutritional software from your smartphone, such as SuperTracker and Cronometer.

12 - Links to Resources & The Fight To Change An Industry

In this chapter we will talk about some of the brave people who are in the trenches (so to speak), fighting the battle against the American diet on a day to day basis. At the end of the chapter is a list of books for further reading, and links to further information sources.

The fight to change an industry

Welcome to the battle. On the one side are the entrenched defenders of the American diet. This includes the processed food industry, the meat and dairy industries, and the people who are resistant to change and want to keep their favorite foods and habits at all costs. On the opposing side are small group of doctors, scientists and researchers who have the strength, integrity and determination to face off with the powerful opposing industries. In the middle is the medical establishment who does not want to be perceived as supporting the American diet which would go against their reputation, but who won't take a stand to oppose it because they are making so much money from the health problems caused by it.

Also against the American diet is a growing group of people who want good long term health, and want to be free from food and medical industries that only seek to profit at everyone's expense. Some of these people are average people who have adopted a healthy diet and lifestyle, others are entrepreneurs who are involved in organic farming, community driven agriculture or other health related businesses.

Which side are you on? If you have been on the wrong side it is never too late to switch sides. The entrenched beneficiaries of the standard American diet will defend their profits through deception, promoting confusion and any other means possible. The rank and file in these industries may not know or understand the extent of the problem, but the executives know well what they are doing. This was proven in the tobacco industry when top executives lied to the courts and lied to congress about their direct knowledge and involvement in formulating cigarettes for maximum addiction and about directly targeting advertising at children.

One way that you can join the fight is by not supporting the processed food and factory farmed animal products industries with your money. Vote with your dollars and completely stop buying their products. Support organic farming and community driven agriculture. Apply political pressure if you are able. Teach other people. Join forces with other like minded people. Help to reform school lunches. There are many ways that you can help to turn this around.

This book is built on the foundation set by many fine researchers, doctors and scientists such as Michael Greger, M.D., Joel Fuhrman M. D., Caldwell B. Esselstyn. Jr. M.D., Colin Campbell PhD., Neal Barnard M.D., John A. McDougall M.D., Dean Ornish M.D., Michael Klaper M.D., Terry Shintani M.D., William Harris M.D., Milton Mills, M.D.

and many others. These people have placed their integrity and desire to do what is right over their career prospects and have often received the wrath of the medical establishment and the food industry. We need to support these brave people and encourage more to step forward. Several hundred years ago they would surely have been discredited, imprisoned and possibly executed for stepping forward and going against the establishment in this manner.

Recommended books for further reading

Most of these books are written by top notch research scientists and renowned doctors who have independently come to the conclusion that a whole food diet is superior.

Nutrition and diet

- The End of Dieting - by Joel Fuhrman M. D. There are several other books written by Dr. Fuhrman such as Eat to Live and Super Immunity. I recommend End of Dieting, because it has basically the same information as Eat to Live, but in a clearer and better organized format. Eat to Live is a good book, but most people find it more difficult to read. Dr. Fuhrman goes into detail about the specific health problems caused by animal products and processed foods and tells about the health benefits of many types of whole foods. Dr. Fuhrmans website: http://www.drfuhrman.com/

- Prevent and Reverse Heart Disease - by Caldwell B. Esselstyn. Jr. M.D. Details the advantages of a whole food diet in preventing and reversing heart disease. Dr. Esselstyn is a renowned heart surgeon. Dr. Esselstyn's web site: http://www.dresselstyn.com/site/

- Whole - by T. Colin Campbell PhD. This book talks about why important research findings in the area of nutrition are ignored by the food industry and our society. Dr. Campbell is one of the top nutritional research scientists in the world and has done highly acclaimed peer-reviewed research, such as spearheading the China-Cornell-Oxford project. Dr. Campbell's website: http://nutritionstudies.org/

- The China Study - by T. Colin Campbell PhD and Thomas M. Campbell II. This book summarizes the China-Cornell-Oxford Project (China Study) that is cited in chapter four.

- The Starch Solution - John A. McDougall M.D. I was put off by the name of this book and put off reading it for a long time, but it is a good book. This doctor tells first hand about the effect the American diet had on his patients and the improvements he observed when they switch to a whole food diet. Dr. McDougall's web site: https://www.drmcdougall.com/index.php

- Dr. Neal Barnard's Program for Reversing Diabetes - by Neal Barnard M.D. This book shows how to reverse type 2 diabetes without drugs, by rejecting the

American diet. Backed by studies funded by the National Institute of Health. Dr.l Barnard's website: http://www.nealbarnard.org/

- Rethink Food: 100+ Doctors Can't Be Wrong - by Shushana Castle and Amy-Lee Goodman. This book has interviews with over 100 doctors advocating a whole food diet.

- Diet Cults: The Surprising Fallacy at the Core of Nutrition Fads and a Guide to Healthy Eating for the Rest of US - In this book Matt Fitzgerald talks about why people are so polarized when it comes to diet and nutrition. I don't agree with all of his opinions about what constitutes a good diet, the important thing is that this book provides food for thought in an area that badly needs more research.

- Forks Over Knives - by Gene Stone. This book features the work of several doctors and researchers, it advocates a plant based diet in an easy to understand style.

- The Happy Herbivore Guide to Plant-Based Living - by Lindsay Nixon. The whole food diet from the perspective of a popular chef.

- The Engine 2 Diet - by Rip Esselstyn. This is a popular diet book promoting a whole food plant based diet.

- Pandora's Lunchbox - by Melanie Warner. An illuminating and detailed look at the food industry and processed food.

Food & Cooking

- The Moosewood Restaurant Cooking for Health - by Moosewood Collective. The healthiest book from the Moosewood folks, who have many popular cookbooks in print.

- Veganomicon: The Ultimate Vegan Cookbook - Isa Chandra Moskowitz and Terry Hope Romero. This book is great for ideas, some of the recipes have to be modified to remove unwanted ingredients such as oil.

- Isa Does It: Amazingly Easy, Wildly Delicious Vegan Recipes for Every Day of the Week Hardcover – Isa Chandra Moskowitz. This book is great for ideas, some of the recipes have to be modified to remove unwanted ingredients.

- Happy Herbivore Light & Lean: Over 150 Low-Calorie Recipes with Workout Plans for Looking and Feeling Great - Lindsay S. Nixon

- The Oh She Glows Cookbook: Over 100 Vegan Recipes to Glow from the Inside Out - Angela Liddon

- Healthy Bread in Five Minutes a Day: 100 New Recipes Featuring Whole Grains, Fruits, Vegetables, and Gluten-Free Ingredients - Zoe Francois, Jeff Hertzberg M.D.

- Wild Fermentation: The Flavor, Nutrition, and Craft of Live-Culture Foods Reclaiming Domesticity from a Consumer Culture - Sandor Ellix Katz

- The Art of Fermentation: An In-Depth Exploration of Essential Concepts and Processes from around the World - Sandor Ellix Katz.

- The Dehydrator Bible: Includes over 400 Recipes - Jennifer MacKenzie, Jay Nutt, Don Mercer.

- Eating on the Wild Side - by Jo Robinson. Most varieties of fruits and vegetables available in stores were domesticated (bred) from wild varieties thousands of years ago. If you are curious about the effects of breeding and want to compare the original and domesticated varieties, this is a good book.

- Edible Wild Plants - by John Kallas PhD. This is a good place to start if you are thinking about foraging and eating wild plants.

Food psychology & breaking food addictions

- Breaking the Food Seduction: The Hidden Reasons Behind Food Cravings---And 7 Steps to End Them Naturally - Neal D. Barnard M.D. This book covers the chemical and biological underpinnings of food addictions and explains how to break food addictions.

- The Pleasure Trap - by Douglas J. Lisle. Goes into detail about food psychology. Also covers methods of overcoming food addictions.

Paleoethnobotany & historical perspectives on the human diet

- Method and Theory in Paleoethnobotany Paperback – John M. Marston (Editor), Jade d'Alpoim Guedes (Editor), Christina Warinner (Editor) This book covers advances in paleoethnobotany including ancient DNA, stable isotope analysis, starch grain analysis, digital data management, and ecological and post processual theory.

Recommended videos

Videos are a good way to learn about diet and nutrition and are more relaxing and easier to digest than reading for most people. One advantage to videos is that you get to see the presenters and get a sense of who they are and how they got involved in promoting healthy eating. Videos are great for getting through to family members who may not want to take the time to read an entire book. Videos that are on Youtube and at other sites can have their locations changed from time to time. If the following links no longer work, do a search on Youtube or google to try to find the new location.

- Uprooting the Leading Causes of Death - Michael Greger M.D. In this video Dr. Greger goes over causes of death with a lot of insight on how the government and medical industries are not addressing these problems. It also shows how a plant based diet addresses the same diseases. https://www.youtube.com/watch?v=30gEiweaAVQ

- Chocolate, Cheese, Meat, and Sugar -- Physically Addictive - Neal Barnard M.D. This video goes over the science behind addictive foods. This is one of the clearest presentations on this subject I have seen, a must see for anyone changing their diet or trying to break food addictions. https://www.youtube.com/watch?v=5VWi6dXCT7I

- Forks Over Knives DVD - Features appearances from several speakers. This DVD is a great way to convey the virtues of a plant based diet in an easy to watch video format. It is available through Amazon.com and other book sellers and may be available through on-demand video providers.

- Dean Ornish: Healing through diet - Dean Ornish M.D. gives a TED talk about the body's natural ability to heal itself. http://www.ted.com/talks/dean_ornish_on_healing Dr. Ornish's website: http://deanornish.com/

- I Love Nutritional Science: Dr. Joel Fuhrman at TEDxCharlottesville 2013 https://www.youtube.com/watch?v=E4katnfHzXA

- Plant-strong & healthy living: Rip Esselstyn at TEDxFremont. Rip is author of The Engine 2 Diet, and talks about several subjects including how the American diet causes erectitle disfunction (ED) https://www.youtube.com/watch?v=AAkEYcmCCCk

- Fine Tuning Your Vegan Diet - William Harris, M.D. In this video Dr. Harris brings up a lot of interesting details about nutrients. https://www.youtube.com/watch?v=JDJpkBoUrrM

- The Ultimate Diet Therapy - Youtube video by John McDougall, M.D. This video dissects and exposes the pseudo science behind the Grain Brain and Wheat Belly fad diets and shows how these diets are just repackaged newer versions of the Atkins diet. https://www.youtube.com/watch?v=kOfF_r2R8QM

- Are Humans Designed To Eat Meat? Dr. Milton Mills, M.D. Goes over the anatomical differences between carnivores and herbivores in great detail. https://www.youtube.com/watch?v=sH-hs2v-UjI

- What's wrong with what we eat - New York Times food writer Mark Bittman gives a TED talk about the American diet. http://www.ted.com/talks/mark_bittman_on_what_s_wrong_with_what_we_eat

- Restaurant Food & Olive Oil Is Not Healthy - YouTube video by Michael Klaper M.D. https://www.youtube.com/watch?v=OGGQxJLuVjg

- What's the Healthiest Diet? - This is an interesting debate between some of the top people advocating whole food diets, they argue about if starches or green and yellow vegetables should be emphasized more. https://www.youtube.com/watch?v=mdxVfi632Xw

- Food That Kills - Full Documentary - YouTube video by Michael Klaper M.D. This video is from 1993, but is just as relevant today as it was then. It shows the health impacts of the American diet, specifically it shows what fat looks like in the blood and what clogged arteries look like. The video may change location on Youtube, search for it if this link doesn't work, it is worth searching to find it. At the present time the video can be found at this link: https://www.youtube.com/watch?v=KNCGkprGW_o Another similar but more modern video from Dr. Klaper: https://www.youtube.com/watch?v=KatsJk0oBUI Dr. Klaper has additional videos that may be of interest on his site: http://doctorklaper.com/videos/

- Debunking the paleo diet - Christina Warinner is a pioneer in biomolecular investigation of archaeological dental calculus (tartar) to study long-term trends in the human diet. She specializes in ancient DNA analysis and paleodietary reconstruction. https://www.youtube.com/watch?v=BMOjVYgYaG8

Recommended websites

Wikipedia

Wikipedia is a great resource, most of the information on Wikipedia is of excellent quality, but like any other source you need to make sure that what you are reading makes sense to you. More than outright inaccurate information (which is very rare), I have noticed omissions on Wikipedia. I think that they are susceptible to lawsuits from special interests, sometimes information that is damaging to companies and industries just disappears, with no trace in the dispute resolution logs. That said, for main steam learning, Wikipedia can't be beat and its coverage of scientific subjects like nutrition, foods and metabolism keeps getting better and better.

- http://en.wikibooks.org/wiki/Category:Recipes
- http://en.wikibooks.org/wiki/Category:Cookbook
- http://en.wikipedia.org/wiki/Nutrition
- http://en.wikipedia.org/wiki/Human_nutrition
- http://en.wikipedia.org/wiki/Vegan_nutrition
- http://en.wikipedia.org/wiki/Dietary_Reference_Intake
- http://en.wikipedia.org/wiki/Nutritional_genomics
- http://en.wikipedia.org/wiki/Western_pattern_diet

- http://en.wikipedia.org/wiki/High-intensity_interval_training
- http://en.wikipedia.org/wiki/Food_composition_data
- http://en.wikipedia.org/wiki/List_of_foods
- http://en.wikipedia.org/wiki/List_of_companion_plants

Other sites

- Nutritionfacts.org is a non-commercial, science-based site by Michael Greger, M.D., launched with support by the Jesse & Julie Rasch Foundation. NutritionFacts.org provides the latest nutrition research in bite-sized videos. There are videos on more than a thousand topics, with new videos every day. http://nutritionfacts.org/

- US military technical bulletin TBmed507 about salt and hydration requirements for strenuous exercise and exercise in extreme hot weather - http://armypubs.army.mil/med/dr_pubs/dr_a/pdf/tbmed507.pdf

- US National Institute of Health - Online library resources. This site is great for doing research. http://www.nih.gov/science/library.html

- PUBMED - Another great site for doing research. http://www.ncbi.nlm.nih.gov/pubmed

- Wikipedia entry that tells about PUBMED http://en.wikipedia.org/wiki/PubMed

- Concept2 rowing machine - http://www.concept2.com/

- Vegetarian Society of Hawaii - http://www.vsh.org/

- USDA Interactive DRI Tool - http://fnic.nal.usda.gov/fnic/interactiveDRI/

Environmental Working Group

- Environmental working group - http://www.ewg.org/ You can read about the EWG: http://en.wikipedia.org/wiki/Environmental_Working_Group

- The EWG Dirty Dozen and Clean fifteen - http://www.ewg.org/foodnews/

- The EWG anual rating of conventional foods - http://www.ewg.org/foodnews/summary.php

Fish safety

- http://www.nrdc.org/health/effects/mercury/guide.asp
- http://www.fda.gov/food/foodborneillnesscontaminants/metals/ucm115644.htm
- http://seafood.edf.org/seafood-health-alerts

Large scale studies & health data

The following are links to sites where the large scale studies and country by country data presented in chapter four can be found. You can read the findings and in some cases the entire datasets can be downloaded if you want to review the data yourself.

World Health Organization

- http://www.who.int/healthinfo/statistics/en/
- http://www.who.int/healthinfo/sage/en/
- http://www.who.int/mediacentre/factsheets/fs310/en/
- http://www.who.int/healthinfo/global_burden_disease/GlobalHealthRisks_report_full.pdf?ua=1
- http://www.who.int/healthinfo/global_burden_disease/GBD_report_2004update_full.pdf?ua=1

EPIC Study

- http://epic.iarc.fr/
- http://www.epic-oxford.org/introduction/
- http://en.wikipedia.org/wiki/European_Prospective_Investigation_into_Cancer_and_Nutrition

The China-Cornell-Oxford Project (China Study)

- http://en.wikipedia.org/wiki/China%E2%80%93Cornell%E2%80%93Oxford_Project
- http://www.ctsu.ox.ac.uk/~china/monograph/
- http://aje.oxfordjournals.org/content/135/10/1180.full.pdf+html
- http://web.archive.org/web/20090223222003/http://www.nutrition.cornell.edu/ChinaProject/
- http://nutritionstudies.org/china-study-references/

Frequently Asked Questions

Question: What are your thoughts on credentials and quality of research?

Answer: Some people look for distinguished titles or medical degrees to establish credibility. Unfortunately in this day and age when you can find highly credentialed people on both sides of most major issues, looking for degrees and other titles is not enough. Money interests often control credentialed people, causing them to take any position imaginable. We live in a corrupt world. Quality of research is just as important as credentials.

Who determines what is quality research? We do! We all bear this responsibility. When we blindly trust other people, even when they have lofty credentials we will eventually pay the price. What I have done in this book is to collect and explain research from many sources, such as the sources listed in this chapter.

You should not depend on credentials. You should read enough to recognize who is making sense and who is not. Start digging and answering questions. It is your right and your responsibility. While a PHD would be beneficial if you are going to design and conduct large scale scientific studies, a PHD is not needed to read these studies.

You should go to PUBMED, the NIH or Wikipedia and start reading, learning and asking questions! All of the information that you find may not agree. You may have to spend hours to get a clear idea of what is going on, but you will be glad that you did. If you are really having trouble understanding complex research you can show the research to your doctor a specialist in the particular field and see if they will take the time to go over it with you. You can even try to contact the scientists or researchers that conducted the research or studies directly and ask them questions. I was surprised to find how many researchers were available by email or by phone and were happy to answer my questions about their work.

The books that are listed in this chapter have extensive references to the research on PUBMED and NIH (National Institute of Health). You can use the search facilities of these sites to do your own searches. The health organizations in the EU member countries also have similar sites in many different languages. Unlike 50 years ago when you would have had to spend months in a major medical research library far from home, you can now pull up a tremendous amount of research with a few mouse clicks. There is no reason to be beholden to the talking heads on TV that are feeding you information you have no way of checking!

Unfortunately you can't use Google or other common search engines because you will come up with corporate advertising, shysters and garbage. A simple internet search will give you mostly a selection of people trying to sell you something. A simple internet search will rarely result in credible peer reviewed research or real science-based information.

Wikipedia has some extremely good information, but keep in mind that not everything on Wikipedia can be trusted 100% of the time. This is even true for PUBMED and NIH! You must look at the references on the bottom of the pages to see where the information is coming from and then read some of the referenced studies and documents to determine if you feel they are credible. Try to determine who is paying for the research. You may have to do additional digging.

As new work is done in the fields of diet, health and nutrition we will continue to learn and adapt together. Our knowledge is a living and dynamic thing that should be continually expanding.

13 - Jumpstart Meal Plans

The meal plans presented in this chapter can be used as a starting point for your transition to a whole food diet, or for rapid weight loss. If you have a medical condition or are taking medication please consult your doctor before making any change to your diet. This book is not meant to substitute for medical advice from your doctor.

Using the meal plans

The meal plans are nutritionally balanced and provide the FDA RDI (required daily intake) of vitamins and minerals so you can use them for as long as you like without worrying about a deficiency of vitamins and minerals. This allows you to drop weight rapidly and improve your health at the same time. In contrast, common fad diets are not nutritionally complete and will result in malnutrition or force you to take supplements.

Adjusting the calories

Normal recommended calorie intake for most people is from 1800 to 2400 calories per day. For rapid weight loss you can start with plan A or plan B that have 1100 calories per day. If you are not trying to lose weight you can start with plan A+ or plan B+ in which case we simply add additional foods to plan A or plan B to give us between 1200 to 2400 calories per day.

Rotating between plans

You can rotate between plans on a daily basis to add variety to your diet. Some people like to rotate between plans giving several days of rapid weight loss followed by a higher calorie day.

Substitution of ingredients

The substitutions listed for each meal plan can be used with little or no effect on the nutritional balance or daily requirements. Reasons to use substitutions are: if you don't like some of the foods, you have allergies or you want to add variation if you become bored. If you are using the A or B plans that have 1100 calories per day and want to try other substitutions of foods that are not listed you may want use nutritional software such as Cronometer or Supertracker to see what the impact on the daily nutritional requirements will be.

For more information about Cronometer and Supertracker, see chapter 11. To modify a meal plan using this software first enter the food list and quantities into the software, then add or delete foods, change quantities or make substitutions. The software will automatically calculate the nutritional value and total calories as you make changes. Both Cronometer and Supertracker offer an online help system.

Avoid sugar or sweeteners

Avoid using sugar or other sweeteners, including artificial sweeteners. Any sweeteners will impede your ability to lose weight and hurt the nutritional integrity of the plan. Sugar and sweeteners are processed foods, you can read about the negative health effect of processed food in chapter 2.

Cooking VS raw

Notice that most or all of the ingredients in lunch and dinner for these meal plans are cooked. This is because most people who are transitioning to a whole food diet do not have the required microbes in their digestive system to handle large amounts of raw vegetables. Over time the proper microbes will develop. If you think that you can handle it, you can use the ingredients uncooked to make salads or smoothies. Make sure to wash everything well and go back to cooking for a while if you start to experience digestive problems.

Cooking times

It is important not to overcook. Overcooking will destroy the nutritional value of most foods. Lightly cooking will retain most of the nutritional value and in some cases the nutritional value will actually increase. See chapter 7 for detailed cooking instructions.

Plan A - 1100 calories

Plan A is an aggressive plan that can be used for maximum weight loss. It uses only plant based whole foods. To achieve a nutritionally balanced plan with plant based ingredients required a lot of spinach. Some people may like this, others may not. Natural seasoning will go a long way with plan A, you should experiment until your meals are seasoned the way you like them. Make sure you do not add more salt than is required and check that you are not using seasonings with extra salt in them. This plan already gives you 1800 mg of sodium per day.

   To keep plan A simple, fortified soy milk is used to meet the vitamin D and vitamin B12 requirements. If for some reason you do not want to use fortified soy milk you can substitute fortified almond milk instead. Alternatively you can use water instead of milk and take vitamin D and vitamin B12 each day. To learn more about vitamin D and B12, see the section "Special Considerations" in chapter 4. The single Brazil nut may seem strange, it is there to provide the daily requirement for selenium.

Breakfast:

- 1/2 cup - Oatmeal (whole oats or quick oats)
- 2 cup - Soymilk fortified with vitamins A and D
- 1 Nut - Brazilnuts, dried, unblanched
- 1/3 cup - Walnuts, chopped

- 1 - Banana, raw medium sized (7" to 7-7/8" long)

You can make breakfast as hot oatmeal with walnuts and sliced banana on top, alternatively you can make a breakfast smoothie by putting all of the ingredients into a blender (you may need to add l little water to adjust the consistency). Add cinnamon or other natural flavoring to the hot oatmeal or the smoothie as needed. After you made the oatmeal and did not use the full two cups of soy milk, make sure to drink what is left over!

Lunch:

- 1-1/2 cup - Broccoli, cooked, boiled, drained, without salt
- 1-1/2 cup - Spinach, cooked from fresh, without salt
- 1/2 cup - Peas, green, frozen, cooked, boiled, drained, without salt
- 1/2 cup - Mushrooms, cooked from fresh
- 1 g - Salt, iodized, added to your plate after cooking

There are several ways to prepare lunch in plan A. You can make a vegetable plate. In this case you can stir fry everything instead of boiling, including the broccoli, or you can cook each item separately. Another idea is to put it all in the blender or food processor and make soup or stew (depending on how much you blend it). Last but not least is the green smoothie. In this case you can add a banana or some strawberries if you can tolerate an additional 100 calories.

Dinner:

- 1-1/2 cup - Broccoli, cooked, boiled, drained, without salt
- 1-1/2 cup - Spinach, cooked from fresh, without salt
- 1/2 cup - Peas, green, frozen, cooked, boiled, drained, without salt
- 1/2 cup - Mushrooms, cooked from fresh
- 1 g - Salt, iodized, added to your plate after cooking

Lunch and dinner have the same ingredients. This allows you to prepare them at the same time if you desire. Lunch could be made into a smoothie and dinner could be heated up and eaten as soup or stew. Alternatively you can move some of the ingredients between lunch and dinner if you want the meals to be different.

Substitutions:

- Instead of Broccoli use Collard greens, Brussels sprouts or Kale
- Instead of Oatmeal use Brown rice
- Instead of Peas use Lentils, Lima beans or Black beans

Plan B - 1100 calories

Plan B is an aggressive plan that can be used for maximum weight loss. It includes sardines as a source of vitamin A, vitamin B12 and Omega 3. Natural seasoning will go a long way with plan B, you should experiment until your meals are seasoned the way you like them. Make sure you do not add more salt than is required, check that you are not using seasonings with extra salt in them. This plan already gives you 1800 mg of sodium per day.

Breakfast:

- 1/2 cup - Oatmeal (whole oats or quick oats)
- 1.5 oz - Almonds, unsalted
- 1 - Banana, raw medium sized (7" to 7-7/8" long)
- 1 cup - Water
- 0.5 g - Salt, iodized, added to your plate after cooking

You can be make breakfast as hot oatmeal with almonds and sliced banana on top, alternatively you can make a breakfast smoothie by putting all of the ingredients into a blender. Add cinnamon or other natural flavoring to the hot oatmeal or the smoothie as needed.

Lunch:

- 1 cup - Turnip greens, cooked from fresh, without salt
- 1 cup - Spinach, cooked from fresh, without salt
- 1/2 cup - Peas, green, frozen, cooked, boiled, drained, without salt
- 1/2 cup - Mushrooms, cooked from fresh
- 1 tbsp - Peanut Butter, without salt
- 1.5 oz - Sardines, canned in water, drained
- 1 g - Salt, iodized, added to your plate after cooking

There are several ways to prepare lunch in plan B. You can make a vegetable plate. In this case you can stir fry everything, or you can cook each item separately. The peanut butter can be mixed with vinegar to make peanut vinaigrette sauce or you can just eat the peanut butter from the spoon. Make sure to use natural peanut butter (with no added oils or other unwanted ingredients). Another idea is to put it all in the blender or food processor and make soup or stew (depending on how much you blend it). Last but not least is the green smoothie. In this case you can add a banana or some strawberries if you can tolerate an additional 100 calories.

Dinner:

- 1 cup - Turnip greens, cooked from fresh, without salt
- 1 cup - Spinach, cooked from fresh, without salt
- 1/2 cup - Peas, green, frozen, cooked, boiled, drained, without salt
- 1/2 cup - Mushrooms, cooked from fresh
- 1 tbsp - Peanut Butter, without salt
- 1.5 oz - Sardines, canned in water, drained
- 1 g - Salt, iodized, added to your plate after cooking

Lunch and dinner have the same ingredients. This allows you to prepare them at the same time if you desire. Lunch could be made into a smoothie and dinner could be heated up and eaten as soup or stew. Alternatively you can move some of the ingredients between lunch and dinner if you want the meals to be different.

Substitutions:

- Instead of turnip greens use Collard greens, Brussels sprouts, Kale or broccoli
- Instead of Oatmeal use Brown rice
- Instead of Peas use Lentils, Lima beans or Black beans

Plan A+ and Plan B+ 1200-2400 calories

In the plus plans we use plan A or plan B as a nutritional foundation and add additional food. If you are trying to lose weight you can count the added calories of the additional food and add it to the base plan to find your total calories. If you are not trying to lose weight you can just add whole foods to plan A or B as you desire without worrying about the calories. The advantage of using plans A or B as a foundation is that you are already starting with a nutritionally balanced diet that provides your recommended daily requirements of vitamins and minerals. This jumpstarts your transition to a whole food diet.

Selecting the additional foods for plan A+ or B+ is easy. In chapter 6 is a master list of all whole foods that are readily available in most stores. You can read chapter 7 for ideas about cooking and preparation. Chapters 8 and 9 have side dishes and meals for breakfast lunch and dinner.

Frequently Asked Questions

Question: I notice that in plan A there is no meat or animal products of any kind. How can this be healthy with no protein?

Answer: Plan A does provide protein, in fact it has 63 grams which is 116% of the recommended daily requirement for adults in the US. The idea that vegetables or other plant based foods do not have protein is a common misconception. I am always surprised by how many people think that meat is protein. Meat has protein in it, but so do vegetables. In fact the protein in plant based foods is superior to the protein in meat because plant based foods do not promote cancer and heart disease.

Question: How were these meal plans calculated and what nutrients to they include?

Answer: The meal plans were calculated using Cronometer nutrition software and the USDA National Nutrient Database for Standard Reference SR27. The meal plans provide the daily requirement for adults in the US of the following nutrients: Protein, Carbohydrates, Lipids, Omega-3, Omega-6, Cystine, Histidine, Isoleucine, Leucine, Lysine, Vitamin B1 (Thiamine), Vitamin B12 (Cobalamin), Vitamin B2 (Riboflavin), Vitamin B3 (Niacin), Vitamin B5 (Pantothenic Acid), Vitamin B6 (Pyridoxine), Folate, Vitamin A, Vitamin C, Vitamin D, Vitamin E, Vitamin K, Calcium, Copper, Iron, Magnesium, Manganese, Phosphorus, Potassium, Selenium, Sodium, Zinc, Methionine, Phenylalanine, Threonine, Tryptophan, Tyrosine, Valine.

Made in the USA
San Bernardino, CA
02 March 2015